HOW TO REDUCE YOUR RISK OF BREAST CANCER

JON J. MICHNOVICZ, M.D., PH.D.
AND DIANE S. KLEIN

WARNER BOOKS

A Time Warner Company

This book describes a preventive approach to disease. It is not meant as a substitute for the medical advice of your personal physician. All women and men should regularly consult a physician in matters relating to their health. This is particularly true for any symptoms of breast disease that may require diagnosis or prompt medical attention. Readers are advised to consult with their physicians before beginning any program of nutritional or dietary change.

Warner Books, Inc., 1271 Avenue of the Americas, New York, NY 10020

 A Time Warner Company

Printed in the United States of America
First Printing: July 1994
10 9 8 7 6 5 4 3 2 1

Library of Congress Cataloging-in-Publication Data

Michnovicz, Jon J.
　　How to reduce your risk of breast cancer / by Jon J. Michnovicz
and Diane S. Klein
　　　　p.　　cm.
　　Includes bibliographical references and index.
　　ISBN 0-446-51751-8 :
　　1. Breast—Cancer—Prevention.　2. Breast—Cancer—Risk factors.
I. Klein, Diane.　II. Title.
RC280.B8M49　1994
616.99′449052—dc20　　　　　　　　　　　　　　　93-41191
　　　　　　　　　　　　　　　　　　　　　　　　　　CIP

Book design by Giorgetta Bell McRee

To every woman struggling to realize the dream of cancer prevention—we offer this book as a gift of empowerment and hope.

_____

To all the women in my life, my mother, my sisters, and especially my wife Stephanie, and our expected child.

J.J.M.

_____

And to my daughters, Beverly and Carolyn, and my baby granddaughters.

D.S.K.

CONTENTS

We wish to thank Frank Cosentino for his invaluable help in the conception and realization of this project.

ACKNOWLEDGMENTS ──────────────────

I would like to thank my colleagues for taking the time from their busy schedules to review the manuscript of this book. Drs. Paolo Toniolo and Ronald Blum at the New York University Medical Center deserve special acknowledgment for their personal encouragement and their professional commitment to cancer prevention research.

I am also grateful to Kara Smigel of the National Cancer Institute's Office of Cancer Communication for her help in providing many useful documents. The staff of the Center for Science in the Public Interest in Washington, D.C., also deserve acknowledgment for their cheerful help in gathering important nutritional information for this book.

J.J.M.

I am particularly grateful to my husband, Elliott, whose understanding, patience, and insight are deeply appreciated. In addition, I am indebted to a good friend, Karen Keen, who graciously shared some of her own wonderful recipes. I wish to thank my sons-in-law, Francisco R. Cuevas, for his invaluable research into America's eating habits, and Andrew E. Lituchy, M.D., for his critical review of this book.

I wish to thank John Paino, President of Nasoya, Inc., for generously sharing several tofu-based recipes. In addition, I am indebted to the following individuals for their help in my research: Linda Meyers of the U.S. Public Health Service; Nancy Volker, Shari Vott and Frank Mahaney of the NCI's Press Office; and Julie Ann Goldman of the CSPI. To these and many others who helped to bring this project to reality, I owe a debt of gratitude.

D.S.K.

Together we thank our editor, Joann Davis, for her critical review of our manuscript as it evolved. Her suggestions greatly strengthened this book. We thank the staff of Warner Books for their assistance, and our agent Barbara Bova for bringing us all together. Finally, we wish to acknowledge David G. Biozes, administrator of The Foundation for Preventive Oncology, Inc., for his help in producing this book.

FOREWORD

Breast cancer is a cruel disease that strikes women down in their prime. Unfortunately, many current therapies for this disease have side effects that may seem equally cruel.

In my office practice, I see increasing numbers of women who seek help to deal with the effects of treatment. Some come because their body image and their self-confidence have been destroyed by mastectomy. Others come because they simply were not prepared for the premature menopause nor for the damage to their sexual responsiveness brought about by the toxic effects of chemotherapy.

The incidence of breast cancer has been rising inexplicably for decades, to the point where most of us personally know one or more women who have been afflicted. And there is still no cure. Incredible as it seems, the outlook for women whose cancer has advanced beyond the operable stage is no better today than it was sixty years ago. Clearly, our best hope is prevention. Unfortunately, the lion's share of breast cancer funding is still devoted to treatment. Only a minuscule portion of the funds available are devoted to preventive strategies.

Dr. Michnovicz's and Ms. Klein's book is like a breath of fresh air. The authors, one a distinguished cancer researcher and physician, the other a science writer, have written a book on the prevention of breast cancer that explains how ordinary women can significantly reduce their risks now, without waiting for further research, simply by changing their diets.

The therapeutic breast cancer prevention program outlined in this book emphasizes increasing the consumption of fruits and vegetables. Deceptively simple, Dr. Michnovicz's preventive nutritional strategies go beyond simply reducing fat, which is great advice but old hat. The authors explain the scientific basis upon which these strategies and recommendations are based.

How to Reduce Your Risk of Breast Cancer describes the natural anti-cancer substances, or phytochemicals, that are contained in various classes of fruits and vegetables. In simple, nonjargon terms, the authors explain the biological mechanisms by which these agents exert their beneficial effects. The important research on "good" and "bad" estrogen, pioneered by Dr. Michnovicz and his colleagues, is summarized. He reports as well on the latest chemoprevention research from laboratories all over the world.

Dr. Michnovicz, being above all an ethical physician, makes no exaggerated claims that his dietary recommendations will prevent all breast cancers. Rather, he explains why and how adherence to this regimen can be expected to lower a woman's risks. Neither does he suggest that increasing the consumption of natural anti-cancer foods is a substitute for early detection practices, such as breast self-examinations and mammography. In fact, the authors strongly encourage women to continue these practices.

This book offers a risk-free, practical and scientifically valid plan of dietary and lifestyle change which will give women the opportunity to take a pro-active stance toward reducing their risk of contracting this dreaded disease. Instead of standing helplessly in the path of the oncoming epidemic, women can now take positive action and *do something* to protect themselves. At the same time, they can improve the health and nutrition of everyone in their families, men as well as women.

Helen Singer Kaplan, M.D., Ph.D.
Director, Human Sexuality Program
The New York Hospital–Cornell Medical Center
New York City

_____

CHAPTER ONE

FACING THE FACTS ABOUT BREAST CANCER

Introduction

Women are beginning to raise questions about breast cancer that go beyond discussions concerning early detection and treatment. Alarmed by the rising incidence of breast cancer, they ask with ever-growing impatience, "What can I do now to *prevent* breast cancer? Is there anything I can do *today* to reduce my risk?"

The good news is *yes*: There are steps you can take today to lower your risk. Answers to the question of breast cancer prevention are beginning to emerge from research laboratories around the world. Perhaps the most encouraging research discovery is the power of naturally occurring substances in vegetables, fruits, and grains to promote health and prevent disease. This finding can have a greater impact on your health and that of your entire family than you may realize.

Drawing upon the results of decades of research, the National Academy of Sciences announced in 1992: "There is sufficient evidence that consumption of certain vegetables, especially carotene-rich (dark green and deep yellow) vegetables and cruciferous (cabbage family) vegetables is associated with the reductions of cancer in humans." This scientific conclusion has become the basis for a nationwide program sponsored by the U.S. National Cancer Institute (NCI), called Eat More Fruits and Vegetables: Five-a-Day for Better Health. The Five-a-Day program encourages everyone to consume at least five to nine servings of vegetables and fruits *each day*. This book will help you understand how and why these guidelines can protect you and your family from the threat of breast cancer.

It is becoming increasingly clear that women can decrease their breast cancer risk by carefully choosing the foods they eat. Some of the world's most highly regarded research scientists have concluded that dietary factors could play a role in as many as *70 percent* of all cancers, including breast cancer.

Still, some will argue that medical science cannot be so definite in its recommendations. They will insist we simply know too little about the causes of cancer to offer answers at this time. "Perhaps we will know all the facts in ten or fifteen years," they reassure us. "Then we can discuss prevention." By then, however, at least 450,000 *more* American women will have lost their lives to breast cancer.

Women need to understand that this pessimistic attitude is no longer justified. There are dozens of clues about the factors influencing breast cancer rates. As Dr. Edward Sondik of the National Cancer Institute stated in *Cancer Objectives for the Nation: 1985–2000*, "There has been a sense that cancer is a problem we can't get hold of, that we as individuals can't do much about, and that just isn't true."

The key to breast cancer prevention lies in minimizing as many of the individual risk factors as possible. Even a slight reduction in risk could save thousands of lives over time. Of all the possible ways to diminish your risk, *dietary change is the most immediate*. Other approaches to preventing this tragic disease will certainly emerge as research continues. But diet is under *your* direct control. You can make the necessary changes today—you need not wait for tomorrow.

The scientific search for ways to prevent cancer is the focus of a new medical research discipline called preventive oncology. Oncology is the branch of medical science that deals with cancer and its treatment. Preventive oncology refers to the study of cancer prevention, a young science incorporating insights from the fields of epidemiology, clinical nutrition, endocrinology, surgery, molecular biology, and radiology. Preventive oncology seeks to discover ways of forestalling or preventing altogether the development of a malignant tumor.

Most of the concern about reducing breast cancer rates has been focused until now on secondary prevention. These secondary measures seek to detect whether a woman already has a breast tumor, through mammography, frequent breast exams, and biopsies. These measures *save lives*, a fact for which we can all be grateful. Researchers estimate that proper screening techniques have reduced the likelihood a woman will die from a breast tumor by at least 25 percent. This percentage will undoubtedly improve as high-quality mammograms are made available to more women.

As important as these secondary measures are, however, they do not *prevent* breast cancer. They benefit women by detecting a malignant tumor early, when surgical treatment has the best chance to cure. Primary prevention, in contrast, seeks to stop the processes that lead to the formation of cancerous breast cells in the first place. The goal of our book is to provide you with the information necessary to create your own comprehensive program of primary breast cancer prevention.

This book is a collaborative effort. It could not have been written without the commitment and perseverance of Diane S. Klein. As a health writer interested in the links between diet and breast cancer, Diane refused to be put off as one busy researcher after another told her they simply had no time for an interview. When she called the Foundation for Preventive Oncology, I invited her to tour our laboratory and to learn about our research firsthand. As we spoke, it became obvious to both of us that it was time women were brought up to date on the latest scientific findings concerning the reduction of their breast cancer risk.

While over one thousand men develop breast cancer in the United States each year, it is through a woman's experience and perspective that the full impact of breast cancer is felt. Even when she herself is free of the disease, a woman who encounters breast cancer in a relative, friend, or even a stranger may think, Why her and not me?

Throughout this book, Diane and I will speak to you with a single voice. Our goal is to convey to you, clearly and accurately, an understanding of the interactions linking diet, lifestyle, and breast cancer. Each of us brings our own perspective to this task. Diane's point of view is that of a woman *at risk*, and mine that of a physician and researcher dedicated to reducing that risk. Our individual experiences complement each other. However, since the stark reality of breast cancer is most clearly perceived through a woman's eyes, Diane will tell her own story here.

A Woman's Perspective

I was twenty-one years old when I met my future mother-in-law. She was fifty and had undergone a radical mastectomy for breast cancer two years earlier. Unfortunately, within a year the cancer had traveled through her bloodstream to her spine, and she began to have severe back pain. Although she was placed in a number of chemotherapy trials, nothing worked for long.

As newlyweds, my husband and I lived nearby. I watched helplessly, day by day, as a plump, sweet-faced wife and mother gradually deteriorated into a bone-thin, pale woman racked with pain. But it was even more devastating for my husband. He was a young doctor, and he knew nothing could help her except the injections of painkillers he gave as temporary relief from her misery.

My mother-in-law's only wish was to be allowed to die at home, and she begged my father-in-law to promise he would never send her to a hospital. Fortunately, the family was able to hire two compassionate nurses who stayed with her for many weeks after she became completely bedridden. On Christmas morning, at the age of fifty-two, my mother-in-law died in her own bed. Her valiant fight was over.

And even though it happened more than thirty-five years ago, it still seems like yesterday. I remember thinking, When I get to be *her* age, doctors will surely have the answer to breast cancer. Women will no longer have to die like this. Only about one in twenty women were likely to develop breast cancer then. Now, according to the latest government statistics, as many as one in eight women in this country will eventually suffer from this disease.

Why are there so many women with breast cancer today? And why should such a large number of them have to lose their lives to this terrible disease, just like my mother-in-law? In this book, we will address these questions and help each woman to design a comprehensive program for reducing her risk of breast cancer.

What the Statistics Can Tell You About Your Breast Cancer Risk

"The biopsy results are in. I'm sorry I have to tell you that you have breast cancer."

Women will hear few words from their physicians as frightening as these. Unfortunately, this diagnosis is becoming more and more common. Is there anyone who does not know at least one friend, relative, neighbor, or coworker with this illness? Most of us, in fact, are probably acquainted with more than one person who has been diagnosed with breast cancer.

The female breast can signify many things: femininity, nurturing love, beauty, sexuality. Breast cancer, therefore, can threaten not only a woman's physical well-being but also her very sense of self. As a married woman poignantly expressed in a recent letter to "Dear Abby," "A cancerous lump was found in my breast. I do not want that breast removed. To know that I may wake up and find that I am only part of a woman scares me to death."

For many women, the threat of breast cancer has become truly alarming. There is a feeling that cancer rates are climbing relentlessly and that there is little we can do about it. But is this true? Are breast cancer rates really increasing? A careful examination of the statistics reveals a disturbing picture. It is one no woman can afford to ignore.

In 1993, women in the United States learned that new calculations by the NCI revealed one out of every eight of them living past the age of eighty-five could be expected to develop breast cancer. Many women were just coming to grips with the one in nine odds previously announced by the NCI—only to discover their risk was even higher still.

Shortly after this announcement was made, an article published in *The New York Times* described the revision of these statistics as merely the correction of "faulty math." The change in odds, the article argued, did not reflect a true increase in breast cancer rates; rather, the higher tumor rates were simply the result of more women getting regular mammograms.

It is easy to understand how any woman trying to follow this debate in the press and on television could become confused. While some news reports have attempted to reassure women breast cancer is not a growing problem, the sad truth is that the occurrence of breast cancer *is* indeed on the rise in our country and elsewhere around the world.

Breast cancer is the most frequently occurring malignant tumor in American women. It accounts for nearly one-third of all new cancer cases *each year*. The latest government statistics indicate that approximately 180,000 women were newly diagnosed with the disease in 1992, while 46,000 women died the same year. Approximately 126 women die *every day* somewhere in the United States as a direct result of a malignant breast tumor.

The increase in breast cancer cases over the past three decades reveals a startling trend. The following published data tell a depressing story.

YEAR	NEW BREAST CANCER CASES
1961	63,000
1965	63,900
1968	65,000
1970	68,000
1972	70,000
1974	89,000
1976	88,000
1978	90,000
1980	108,000
1982	112,000
1984	115,000
1986	123,000
1988	135,000
1989	142,000
1991	175,000
1992	180,000

Source: Surveillance, Epidemiology, and End Results
(SEER) Program of the National Cancer Institute

These statistics document a frightening increase in the number of women who develop breast cancer. Do these numbers reflect things as they really are? Or does the incidence of breast cancer only *seem* to be rising, a statistical result of the aging and growth of our population?

When computing such statistics, medical researchers make an adjustment for the increased numbers of women in our society. And, since breast cancer occurs most often in older women, researchers also have to allow for the fact that Americans are growing older on average. The scientists use what is called an "age-adjusted" disease rate, which shows the average number of new cases of the disease for every 100,000 women of *all ages* in a given country.

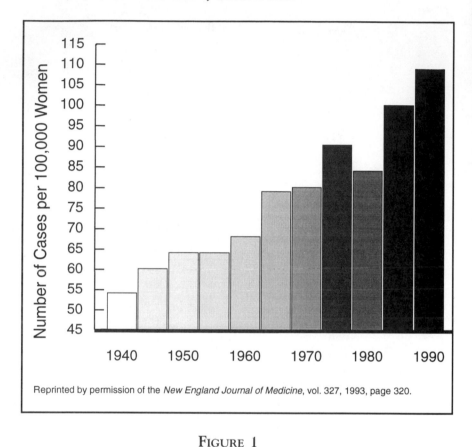

FIGURE 1

Trends in Breast Cancer Rates in the U.S. Over the Past Five Decades

Figure 1 illustrates the age-adjusted disease rates in the United States and makes it obvious that *breast cancer rates are definitely going up*. This increase in risk is no statistical quirk—it is a harsh fact.

Are the increased rates of breast cancer shown in Figure 1 simply the result of early detection due to the increased use of mammography? The answer is *no*, based on two important facts. First, it has been only within the last ten or fifteen years that mammograms have been readily available to many American women.

Breast cancer rates, on the other hand, have been on the rise for several decades. Second, screening mammograms are still vastly underutilized. Only about one-third of the women who could benefit from mammograms actually get them. Increased screening alone cannot account for the steady upward climb in breast cancer rates.

It is true that a small fraction of the increase in new cases of this disease may come from the earlier discovery of smaller tumors in women. Such a statistical effect was indeed recorded in 1974, following the widely publicized cases of breast cancer in Betty Ford and Happy Rockefeller. A higher-than-expected increase in cases was seen that year because so many more women decided to go for a mammogram. Since then, however, cancer rates have continued to escalate.

The conclusion is unavoidable: Cases of breast cancer have been steadily increasing, both here and elsewhere around the world. Consider the recently published data from the World Health Organization, shown in Figure 2. In this report, researchers measured changes over time in breast cancer death rates among women aged thirty-five to sixty-nine living in a number of countries. The upward trends charted in this figure are all too familiar. Breast cancer deaths are rising in countries all over the world. Even in Japan, where the rates are still low, there has been a noticeable increase, as well.

Do medical scientists have any idea why breast cancer rates continue to climb?

Thus far, there is no medical agreement as to the *major* cause of this worldwide increase in breast cancer deaths. As we will see, there are many individual risk factors to consider in breast cancer.

As Figure 2 clearly shows, deaths from malignant breast tumors have been increasing globally over the last thirty years. The death rates in the United States from this illness have not significantly improved, even with our greater use of mammography. After years of research into new methods of chemotherapy, the odds of a woman surviving from this disease are not getting better. Women are frightened, and for good reason.

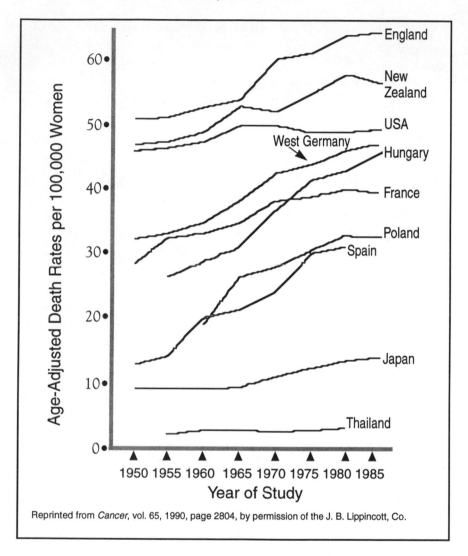

Reprinted from *Cancer*, vol. 65, 1990, page 2804, by permission of the J. B. Lippincott, Co.

FIGURE 2

Recent Changes in Breast Cancer Death Rates Around the World

The Unique Importance of Diet in the Primary Prevention of Breast Cancer

Over the past decade, researchers have begun to understand the basic mechanisms that affect a woman's risk. When a disease is as widespread in the population as breast cancer, positive changes in even one of the minor risk factors can add up to thousands of lives lost or saved. Review the statistics once more: 180,000 American women developed a breast tumor *in 1992 alone.* And this trend shows no signs of reversing. If we had a way to reduce the odds all women face by only 5 percent, as many as nine thousand women would not have to confront the diagnosis of a malignant breast tumor. In fact, some prominent researchers believe the incidence of breast cancer in women could be lowered by *at least 33 percent.*

A reduction in breast cancer risk of 33 percent *this year* alone could spare nearly sixty thousand American women the physical and emotional suffering caused by a malignant breast tumor. Such a reduction would also lower the high medical costs of caring for these women. Multiplied many times around the world, even a small change in risk could have a very great impact on breast cancer deaths.

In the next chapter, beginning on page 27, you will learn that scientists have identified four broad categories of breast cancer risk, each of which includes various contributing factors. The categories are: reproductive; individual and genetic; environmental; and dietary and lifestyle risk factors.

While some of the important risk factors for breast cancer cannot be changed—your age at first menstruation or your family history, for example—some risks *can* be lowered. Diet is one of the categories in which change *is possible.* Unlike any other approach to risk reduction, dietary change meets the following five criteria.

1. *Dietary change is under your direct control.*
   You do not need to depend on anyone else to make this change in your life.

2. *Dietary changes can be enjoyable.*

Gone are the days when healthy eating meant bland food and dull recipes. Low-fat, high vegetable/fruit dishes are easy to prepare. As food manufacturers begin to recognize the enormous market for healthier foods, more and more of these products will find their way to your supermarket shelves.

3. *Dietary changes can be started today.*

There is no need to wait for the results of further government studies on the important link between nutrition and your health. The results are in, and scientists are convinced of the healthful effects of dietary change.

4. *Dietary changes can protect you from a variety of other chronic diseases as well as breast cancer.*

This is a truly remarkable fact. Many scientists are convinced that nutritional changes such as those described in this book are likely to reduce your risk not only for breast cancer but for colon cancer, heart disease, and other chronic illnesses.

5. *Dietary changes you make can protect your daughters and your entire family.*

New dietary habits in the household will positively affect the lives of the entire family.

All of these reasons justify our emphasis on the role of dietary change as a key strategy in an overall program of breast cancer risk reduction. Women can begin right *now* to make the changes necessary to reduce their risk of developing this disease. But do medical researchers know the specific kinds of nutritional changes women need to make to reduce that risk?

The answer is yes: Women need to introduce more vegetables, whole grains, and fruits into their diets. You may be asking yourself, however, if this can really be true. Can such commonplace foods actually make such a difference in breast cancer risk? In the war against cancer, dietary change may seem too feeble a weapon to be of much help. Our purpose here is to explain just how potent a weapon nutrition can be in the effort to reduce breast cancer rates.

One of the main goals of this book is to explain the reasons *why* many researchers have come to believe in the protective benefits of dietary change.

Eat More Fruits and Vegetables: Five-a-Day for Better Health

Medical experts are increasingly convinced that *the general health of the American people would vastly improve if they started to eat more fresh fruits and vegetables daily.* As a result, the National Institutes of Health and the National Cancer Institute have sponsored a nationwide program, entitled Eat More Fruits and Vegetables: Five-a-Day for Better Health. The aim of this program is to educate all of us about the positive role of fruits and vegetables in reducing the risk of most cancers and other serious chronic disorders.

The new program encourages American adults to eat *at least* five half-cup servings of fruits and vegetables every day as part of a low-fat, high-fiber diet. In this book, we will draw upon the insights of this program to help explain which vegetables and fruits are particularly helpful in protecting women against breast cancer.

The NCI's Five-a-Day nutritional program grew out of years of careful research into the eating habits of thousands of women and men. How does the average American diet compare in the light of these recommendations? Not very well. According to a July 1992 press release from the U.S. Public Health Service, "Only 8 percent of Americans believe they should be eating at least 5 servings of fruits and vegetables each day to be healthy."

In fact, few Americans even came close to eating the minimum recommended amount of five servings per day. In a nationwide survey of the eating habits of over eleven thousand American adults, only 9 percent of those interviewed had eaten five servings of fruits and vegetables within the past twenty-four hours. Nearly half of all Americans interviewed said they had no fruit or fruit juice on a given day. Nearly half had eaten only one serving of vegetables the previous day, and in some cases this lone vegetable was french fries!

Instead of the five or more servings we should be getting *each day*, therefore, most of us consider ourselves health-conscious if we eat one or two. You may think you are already eating all of the vegetables you need. But how many servings did you really eat today or yesterday? Did you eat just a few grapes, or simply put a piece of lettuce on your ham and cheese sandwich? Did you use some catsup on your hot dog, or take a few sips of orange juice as you rushed off to work?

Before giving any specific recommendations, let's first summarize what NCI experts say on the subject of serving sizes. According to the official guidelines, a serving size can be defined as a medium-sized piece of fruit, six ounces of 100 percent fruit juice, a cup of raw leafy vegetables, a half cup of cooked vegetables, a half cup of diced fresh fruit, or a quarter cup of dried fruit. Remember, the recommendation is five to nine of these servings *each day*—not each week or each month.

According to Dr. Bernadine Healy, former director of the National Institutes of Health, "The importance of diet in the prevention of major killer diseases like cancer and heart disease is paramount. The Five-a-Day message—to eat five or more servings of fruits and vegetables daily—is positive, easy to carry out, and will not be overturned by the food fad of the next week." Unfortunately, over 140 million Americans are not eating the minimum amounts recommended.

You may hate to admit it, but mom was right when she insisted, "Eat your vegetables. They're good for you." Studies show that children with a habit of eating lots of fruits and vegetables in childhood continue to do so as adults. Fewer than one in five youngsters with very low fruit and vegetable consumption improve their eating habits in adulthood.

Writing in the journal *Nutrition and Cancer*, Dr. Gladys Block at the University of California at Berkeley has argued that if Americans increased their fruit and vegetable consumption, they could gain substantial health benefits. She emphasizes that eating more of these breast-healthy foods could represent a simple strategy to reduce cancer risk in women.

Fighting Breast Cancer: The Estrogen-Phytochemical Connection

The NCI's Five-a-Day for Better Health recommendations offer *general guidelines* for the reduction of cancer in women and men. In a later chapter, we will carefully examine the evidence that led NCI researchers to such a strong conclusion regarding the protective properties of vegetables and fruits. It is the potent action of unique plant compounds, called *phytochemicals*, which we will be discussing in this book, that extend the protective benefits of the Five-a-Day program to breast cancer, as well.

There is a common thread running through many of the breast cancer risk factors. It is the female hormone estrogen. You may be surprised to learn that abnormal estrogen stimulation has been implicated in each of the four broad risk categories—reproductive; individual and genetic; environmental; and dietary/lifestyle.

It was an interest in the relationship between estrogen and breast cancer that drew me into the field of preventive oncology nearly a decade ago as a physician and researcher at The Rockefeller University in New York City. Important medical breakthroughs often come about in totally unexpected ways. My own early studies focused on the hormonal effects of cigarette smoking in women. In 1985, scientists in Boston reported that women who smoked cigarettes faced only half the risk of developing cancer of the endometrium (the lining of the uterus), as compared with nonsmokers. This unusual finding was later confirmed by other researchers, and it led our laboratory group to pose a series of questions.

What is it about smoking, we asked, that reduces the risk for a hormone-dependent endometrial cancer? Could the "smoking effect" also protect women against breast cancer? Was there a way for women to receive the same benefits safely, without exposure to the cancer-causing agents in cigarette smoke? And finally, was there some *chemical substance* in smoke that could be isolated and studied for its cancer-preventive properties?

To answer these questions, my colleagues and I studied the effects of cigarette smoking on estrogen in women. The results of this research were published in the *New England Journal of Medicine* and were widely reported in the news media. Our clinical studies showed that the rates at which estrogen was broken down and eliminated in female smokers was nearly double that of nonsmokers. It was our conclusion that smoking decreased a woman's risk for endometrial cancer because it helped remove estrogen from her body. Having discovered this basic biochemical mechanism, we could begin to search for safe substances in foods, which might have an effect similar to the toxic substances present in tobacco smoke.

Members of our laboratory group at The Rockefeller University had previously determined that estrogen travels in the body in different forms. One form of the hormone was found to be unusually *active* and dangerous, apparently able to damage the genetic material of breast cells. This form of estrogen is called C-16. The term refers to the 16-carbon atom of estrogen, one of two sites where estrogen is normally altered during the breakdown process. Alteration at the other site leads to the formation of C-2 estrogen, an *inactive*, safer form.

We soon became aware that many factors associated with breast cancer protection are linked to increased production in a woman's body of the inactive C-2 estrogens. A woman's breast health seems to be best protected when her body produces less of the active C-16 estrogen and more of the C-2 type.

Transferring our work to the newly established Institute for Hormone Research, now the research branch of The Foundation for Preventive Oncology in New York City, my colleagues and I turned our attention to dietary substances that might also favorably affect the pattern of estrogen breakdown in women (a process called estrogen metabolism). Our goal was to identify dietary factors able to protect against breast and endometrial cancer.

We sought those foods that might have properties similar to the compounds in tobacco smoke, but without the dangerous side effects of smoking. Since most foods can be eaten without adverse effects, we believed we would be able to find a substance or substances in the diet that could safely transform estrogen into the most benign form possible.

Research studies into the effects of food chemicals at the Institute for Hormone Research were conducted as part of the National Cancer Institute's Experimental Foods Program. This five-year, $20.5 million study was organized in 1990 to evaluate carefully the properties of natural foods and plants that might benefit human health. This innovative research program has helped support our search for breast-protective foods.

Our studies under the Experimental Foods Program have focused on the hormonal effects of feeding *licorice root* and *flax seed* to experimental animals. In addition, we have examined the effects of some of these same foods on women participating in our research. These two unusual substances were chosen for study by the NCI scientists largely because they had been used safely around the world for many centuries, often for medicinal purposes.

In addition to licorice root and flax seed, the Experimental Foods Program has been investigating the properties of citrus oil, garlic extracts, umbelliferous vegetables (carrot and parsley family), rosemary, cruciferous vegetables (cabbage and broccoli family), and soybeans. The Experimental Foods Program was and is the first project of its kind. Hopefully, it will represent the federal government's commitment to a growing area of research called nutritional chemoprevention.

Our studies of natural substances in our diet also led us to a chemical substance found in the cruciferous family of vegetables, a compound called *indole-3-carbinol* (I-3-C). The cruciferous family includes such common vegetables as cabbage, broccoli, radishes, cauliflower, and brussels sprouts, as well as such lesser-known ones as broccoli rabe, kale, turnips, watercress, and mustard.

Initial laboratory studies of this compound demonstrated a reduction of breast cancers in mice fed I-3-C. In pilot studies of women taking this compound, my colleagues and I have found that I-3-C increased the rate of inactivation and removal of estrogen.

Our studies have demonstrated that many important breast cancer–fighting substances exist in our diet, which may prove helpful in our fight to reduce women's cancer risks. And I-3-C is only a single promising plant chemical, or phytochemical. Each phytochemical could contribute to the already-healthful effects of a low-fat and high-fiber diet. Taken together, they provide the key for understanding how the national Five-a-Day for Better Health program can extend its protection against breast malignancies.

The hundreds of plant substances we *may* eat every day constitute a kind of "natural pharmacy," assisting our bodies in combating chronic diseases like cancer. Some of these phytochemicals have become widely known to the public through television, magazines, and radio. Consider beta-carotene, for example, a phytochemical abundant in carrots, broccoli, and dozens of other vegetables. Beta-carotene helps the body to form vitamin A, which is essential to the health of our tissues. It is becoming increasingly clear that this phytochemical also protects certain cells against cancer, possibly including breast cancer. Many other phytochemicals may be equally important, although they are not yet as well known.

Indeed, the various phytochemicals we *could be eating* each day appear to provide our bodies with a natural arsenal aimed directly against the cancer process. The vast majority of these biochemicals are derived exclusively from plants and cannot be manufactured in our own bodies. While some of these substances may one day become available to consumers in supplement form, the best strategy for getting plentiful amounts of these cancer-fighting agents is to eat a wide variety of fresh fruits, whole grains, and vegetables.

For years, scientists have debated the relative merits of a low-fat diet in protecting women against breast cancer. By focusing predominantly on fat calories, however, scientists may have lost sight of other important dietary factors. Fat calories and phytochemicals usually occur in opposite amounts in our daily diets. The more fat a woman eats, the greater the likelihood that she is eating relatively few fruits and vegetables. On the other hand, the more fresh plant-based foods a woman consumes, the less appetite there is likely to be for greasy, fat-laden foods.

This book will help you to understand which specific phytochemicals are believed to protect the health of your breasts. We will explain how you can harness this natural pharmacy and why medical scientists believe these plant compounds can protect you. This nutritional protection is available to every woman, regardless of the risks she faces.

In the next chapter, we will carefully examine the known risk factors for breast cancer.

UNDERSTANDING BREAST CANCER RISK FACTORS

In order to understand the risk factors that influence the development of breast tumors, we need first to know how the breasts normally function. Let us begin by reviewing the anatomical structures of the breasts.

The Anatomy of the Breasts

The basic function of the breasts, or mammary glands, is to produce milk for newborn and infant children. These glands help to define us as mammals. While the breasts also play a role in other aspects of a woman's life, such as in sexual arousal, it is the breast's primary function as a milk-producing gland that helps to explain the origin of most breast diseases.

Milk is produced by cells grouped into countless tiny sacs inside the breasts. Clustered together, these tiny sacs form a breast *lobule*. Milk produced deep within the lobule flows through a connection of ducts leading toward the nipples. Several lobules connected to a single large duct constitute a *breast lobe*. About fifteen to twenty of the largest ducts, arranged like spokes of a wheel, enter into the nipple.

Surrounding the breast lobes and lobules is a mass of fat tissue, making up about one-third to two-thirds of the total weight of the breasts in most women. After menopause, much of the normal breast tissue is replaced by fat. The breasts also contain blood vessels, some supporting tissue, and small lymph nodes, mostly near the armpits.

Some cancers begin in the breast cells lining the small milk-producing sacs and lobules deep within the breasts, while others form in one of the many large ducts. For this reason, the two major types of breast cancer are termed *lobular* carcinoma and *ductal* carcinoma. Ductal cancers are far more common, with only about 10 to 15 percent of breast cancers originating in the lobules. Occasionally, a breast tumor appears initially near the nipple, a condition called Paget's disease of the nipple. Even in this case, however, the tumor's site of origin is still the ductal cells of the breast.

What Is Breast Cancer?

Breast malignancies, like all other forms of cancer, are defined by the wildly uncontrolled growth of cells and the eventual spreading of these abnormal cells to other parts of the body. It is important to remember that the cells in a malignant breast tumor were originally "normal," like all of the other cells in the breasts. They become abnormal by a process scientists call *genetic mutation*.

A breast cell can undergo mutations for various reasons. To understand what a mutation is, we must first recognize that all of a cell's genetic material is contained in twenty-three pairs of chromosomes. Each chromosome is actually an extremely long, tightly packed single molecule called DNA. Every time a cell divides in two, these long molecules of DNA must be copied *exactly*. A mutation may occur whenever a chance error is made during the copying process.

Every time a breast cell divides, there is a small chance that an error may be made during copying. The faster a tissue or gland grows, the greater the possibility of a chance mutation. Breast cancer researchers at the University of Southern California have recently described this process in detail. They pointed out that many cancer-causing agents irritate the breast cells. This injury induces the cells to grow and multiply more rapidly. In the process, DNA faces a greater risk of being accidentally miscopied, leading to a mutation.

Researchers believe that at least two mutations in a single breast cell are necessary before that cell's growth is changed permanently from a normal pattern into a malignant one. Also, in rapidly growing cells, a chance mutation may occur in the *wrong location* on the DNA molecule, thus resulting in much more serious consequences than other mutations. For example, cancer researchers have recently come to understand that certain DNA genes have the critical job of restricting the growth and division of cells. These are called *tumor-suppressor genes.* A chance mutation that destroys the normal functioning of one of the tumor-suppressor genes in breast cells would probably cause those cells to grow faster than usual. It would be like a runaway car whose brakes are beginning to fail.

Fortunately, even when a cell's DNA is accidentally damaged, your body has a remarkable system ready to mend it. This system includes DNA repair enzymes, which monitor the twenty-three pairs of chromosomes for abnormal-looking DNA. Medical scientists have estimated that the DNA repair enzymes can normally repair thousands of mutations in the body's cells each day. All of this accidental DNA damage is usually restored to a healthy state. In some individuals, however, breast-cell damage may exceed the body's capacity to repair it.

Some women with a genetic risk of breast cancer may have already inherited one of the two mutations needed to convert a breast cell into a permanently malignant state. Such women are at a higher risk of danger from a second chance mutation in their breasts. Any excessive cell growth caused by estrogen in such high-risk women carries a much greater danger than for the average-risk woman.

A major stimulus encouraging a breast cell to divide is exposure to the hormone estrogen. This is one of the reasons why estrogen is linked to breast cancer and why breast tumors often get their start in younger women, though the cancer may remain silent for years. We will discuss how estrogen is related to cell division and breast cancer in much more detail in Chapter 6.

Breast Lumps Are Not Always Cancerous

Benign breast disease has been called by many names over the years. It is not actually a disease, but, rather, a category of nonmalignant breast conditions, which may include any one of the following: fibrocystic breasts, fibroadenoma, breast cysts, proliferative breast disease, and dysplasia. Fibrocystic breast disease, for example, refers to dense, lumpy, often tender breasts. This condition may affect many young women; it occurs when some of the breast cells lining the lobules or ducts grow slightly faster than normal.

A young woman may occasionally notice a distinct lump in one of her breasts, which seems to disappear after a menstrual cycle, only to reappear again later. Such a nodule is likely to be a cyst. Cysts can usually be drained by a technique known as needle aspiration. After the physician drains the cyst, it usually will not recur. The cells lining a breast cyst are rarely malignant.

Another benign breast lump is called a fibroadenoma. These lumps also generally occur in younger women, and they usually feel round and "rubbery" to the touch. They are painless and are easily moved around under the skin of the breast where they are found. Research has shown there is no added risk to developing breast cancer in a woman with a benign fibroadenoma.

There is a category of benign breast disease, however, which is still the subject of medical debate. It is a condition referred to as dysplasia, or *carcinoma in situ*. In situ tumors are being detected more and more often as efficient mammography machines pick up ever smaller abnormalities in younger women. The problem is that doctors cannot be certain whether these cells will ever develop into a full-blown malignancy of the breast. Because of this doubt, some researchers still prefer to characterize this finding as precancerous, using terms such as *proliferative breast disease* or *dysplasia*. Such abnormal changes, however, place a woman at higher risk for developing a breast cancer later in life.

Who Is Affected by Breast Cancer?

Breast cancer, unfortunately, is an "equal opportunity" disease. From the wives of former Presidents to the poorest of women, millions all over the world have faced and continue to face this dreaded diagnosis. We simply do not yet know what causes renegade breast cells to grow out of control in every woman who develops a malignancy.

Women who develop breast cancer may be young or old, affluent or poor, and from any racial or ethnic background. Consider the following brief vignettes of women who developed a breast malignancy. Each case is uniquely different from the next. Perhaps you may recognize someone you know in these acquaintances of ours. Sadly, this list of neighbors, friends, and relatives could go on and on.

Marika

Marika was the sixth child in a family of Hungarian immigrants. Her parents fled Hungary to prevent the father, Josef, from being inducted into the army during World War I.

Marika married young. Her first child, a son, was stillborn and she later had another baby, a little girl. She eventually divorced her husband when she was in her early fifties and married again. That relationship was also a stressful one, and Marika divorced her second husband after only a few years of marriage.

Her doctor found her breast lump on a routine checkup when she was in her mid-sixties. She had the breast removed after it proved to be malignant. With no recurrence of the cancer, Marika continued to work as a secretary until her death from heart disease at the age of seventy-three.

LuAnne

LuAnne was a very frail young black woman of twenty-eight. She was from a large farm family in Alabama. She had moved to New York at the age of eighteen and began working in a factory that made "some kind of chemical stuff."

She met her husband, Johnny, in the neighborhood where she lived. After five children and years of hard times, LuAnne was diagnosed with breast cancer.

"The doc just told me I have a breast tumor and I'm not goin' to be around very long," she confided, "so I need to place the five kids somewhere."

LuAnne was right. Six months after her children were placed in foster care, LuAnne died of breast cancer. Sadly, she had not known anything about her breast tumor until she was already in an advanced stage and it was too late.

Margot

Margot was the adored only child of German Jewish refugees who emigrated to the United States as teenagers in the early 1920s. Her father, an apprentice butcher in the old country, eventually established himself in a butcher shop in the German section of New York City.

Even after Margot was married and gave birth to her only child, a boy, she and her husband continued to live in her parents' two-family home, with grandma doing all the cooking. Beef, heavily marbled with fat, was proudly served every day, along with rich puddings, sweet cream, and butter pastries. To eat "so well" was a sure sign of success for this immigrant family.

Although Margot had been slim as a young woman, by her mid-thirties she started to put on weight around her waist. Only her slim legs reminded one of the slender young girl she had once been. Shortly after her fifty-third birthday, Margot was terrified when she discovered a lump in her breast. The diagnosis, unfortunately, was breast cancer. She underwent a modified radical mastectomy. Within two years, the cancer had spread; despite chemotherapy, Margot died just before the age of fifty-five. Her grief-stricken mother lived to be eighty-four. There was no known history of breast cancer in the family.

Kathleen

Kathleen is an overweight fifty-five-year-old schoolteacher with a body most doctors would call apple-shaped. Four years ago, she had a breast removed and so did her husband, John. Both Kathleen and John had been diagnosed with breast cancer.

Kathleen and John were operated on by the same breast surgeon and were cautioned to reduce the fat content of their diets drastically. They both admitted to being addicted to high-fat foods, especially ice cream. In fact, each of them used to eat a pint of ice cream almost every night while watching TV. With considerable effort, John lost about sixty-five pounds after the operation.

"We have cut down a lot," Kathleen said with a sigh, "but we still can't do without an occasional ice cream fix. However, our thirty-two-year-old daughter is so petrified of developing breast cancer, she has become a vegetarian."

There is no known family history of breast cancer in this large extended Irish family.

Factors That *Increase* Your Risk

Medical scientists have worked for decades to uncover those factors that influence a woman's risk for a breast tumor. The fact that so many different risks have been identified tells us that the health of the breasts can be affected by nearly all aspects of our lives.

For some women who develop breast cancer, few of the known risk factors listed below seem to apply. While many risk factors have been discovered, *the fact remains that nearly three-fourths of all new breast malignancies occur in women without a particularly strong risk profile.* As the authors of an important article on breast cancer in the *New England Journal of Medicine* recently stated, "The search for modifiable risk factors has not been exhausted and must continue."

The extent of increased risk associated with a certain factor is called its "relative risk." The higher the relative risk, the greater the danger associated with it. Let's look at a simple example.

Medical researchers begin by studying a very large group of women, such as those living in a certain county or state. The researchers then carefully record every case of breast cancer occurring over a period of time—five years, for example. Using a computerized data base, they record dozens of specific traits that describe each of the women in their study. These might include a woman's age, her place of birth, race, body weight, height, number of children, and so on. The list of variables can be extensive.

Next, researchers compare how many cancers occurred in those women with a certain trait with the number of cancers in women without that trait. Take the case of family history. Some women who develop breast cancer in the research study will have other family members with the disease; other women will not. The researchers may find in their large population that there are 250 women with breast cancer who do have a positive family history and only 100 women who do not. The relative risk associated with a woman's family history in this study, therefore, is 250/100, or 2.5. In other words, scientists would judge that women with a family history of breast cancer are about two and a half times more likely to develop the disease.

With each of the risk factors listed in this section, medical scientists were able to study large groups of women, and each time they compared women with a certain trait, such as using oral contraceptives, with women not sharing that trait. For some risk factors (such as height), the researchers compared women on one end of the spectrum (for example, the tallest fifth) with women on the other end (the shortest).

We will now examine the various risk factors individually to learn how each one can influence a woman's odds for developing breast cancer. The known risk factors are summarized in the table on page 30, along with the degree of increased risk (relative risk) from each factor listed in the adjacent column.

Reproductive Risk Factors

Early Menarche

The average age at which young women experience their menarche, or first menstruation, has been declining in industrialized countries for over a century. For most American girls, menstruation currently begins around twelve and a half years of age, although some girls begin menstruating even earlier. By contrast, in China and in other countries with much lower cancer rates, the average onset of menstruation begins closer to age seventeen.

By comparing cancer rates in American women who had their first menstruation before age twelve and a half with rates in women having their first period later in life (beyond age fourteen), researchers were able to measure a relative risk of 1.3 associated with the earlier menstruation.

Late First Birth or No Children

Having a first child past the age of thirty, or having no children at all, places a woman at a higher relative risk for developing breast cancer. For such a woman, the risk increases to nearly double that of a woman who completes a full-term pregnancy before age twenty. Among women who never complete a pregnancy, due to miscarriage or abortion, for example, the risk is also approximately doubled.

The most recent observation of this type comes from a study of

KNOWN RISK FACTORS FOR BREAST CANCER

RISK CATEGORY	EXTENT OF INCREASED RISK
Reproductive Factors	
Early menarche	1.3
Late first birth or no children	1.9
Late menopause	1.5
No breast-feeding	1.2
Individual and Genetic Factors	
Family history of breast cancer	2.5
Benign breast disease	2.5
Age (see page 35)	
Height	1.3
Environmental Factors	
Oral contraceptives	1.5
Estrogen replacement therapy	2.1
Alcohol	2.0
Radiation	1.5
Pesticide exposure	2.0
Lifestyle Factors	
Diet	1.5 or greater
Lack of exercise	1.3
Obesity (over age 50)	1.5

lesbian women conducted in 1992 by Dr. Suzanne Haynes, chief of health education in the NCI's Division of Cancer Prevention and Control. Dr. Haynes's data reveal that lesbian women are about three times more likely than heterosexual women to develop a breast malignancy during their lifetime. Dr. Haynes's unpublished findings were reported to the National Lesbian and Gay Health Foundation's 1992 conference, where she concluded that the additional risk was attributed in large part to the lack of childbearing in this group of women.

Late Menopause

Women who begin menopause later in life have a modest increase in their risk for breast cancer. The average age when menopause occurs in the United States is currently around fifty years of age. When scientists compare women experiencing menopause unusually late in life with those having an earlier than usual menopause, they can detect a relative risk around 1.5 associated with this factor.

Both early menarche and late menopause potentially extend the period of a woman's reproductive life, and this may help to explain why each is associated with elevated risk. A later than average menopause allows the breasts to continue to undergo estrogen stimulation each month, over a longer period of time.

Some women with an early menarche also have an early menopause, suggesting that these two factors, in some individuals, could cancel each other out. Remember: These risk factors have been determined by epidemiologists observing the effects of menarche and menopause within large populations of women.

Breast-Feeding

Earlier clinical studies found that women who did not breast-feed their infants appeared to face a higher risk of breast cancer than women who did. Despite these findings, some doubt has persisted about this association. The matter has been resolved by a definitive study published in 1994, which makes it clear that breast-feeding can protect a woman's breasts to a modest degree.

Individual and Genetic Risk Factors

Family History of Breast Cancer

Breast cancer in Western countries occurs so frequently that having a relative with the disease *does not* automatically mean a woman carries a genetic trait, or an inherited cancer gene. Women in the same family may share many things besides their genes. Often, they share similar diets, a comparable level of affluence, or a common exposure to an unknown environmental factor.

Nevertheless, genetic factors clearly play a role in the lives of *some* women with breast cancer. Statistics indicate that there is increased risk to a woman if she has a first-degree female relative (mother, daughter, sister) who developed the disease. If a woman's mother developed a breast malignancy *early* in life, the risk is greater, and should more than one first-degree relative have breast cancer, the risk is even greater still. A woman's risk is also elevated if someone on her father's side has developed breast cancer.

However, *most women* who develop a breast tumor *do not* have a known family history of breast cancer. According to Professor Henry Lynch, director of the Hereditary Cancer Consultation Center at Creighton University School of Medicine in Omaha, Nebraska, most cases of breast cancer, about 70 percent, are actually *sporadic*, occurring in women with no known family history.

On the other hand, a *familial* breast cancer pattern is found in only approximately 25 percent of women initially seen with a malignant breast tumor. In the familial pattern, a woman knows at least one close female relative (mother, daughter, sister, cousin, grandmother) who had the disease. A woman's risk is also increased if a man in the family develops breast cancer.

In roughly 5 to 7 percent of breast cancer cases, women in multiple generations of a single family may be affected. Dr. Lynch and other researchers have termed this *hereditary* breast cancer.

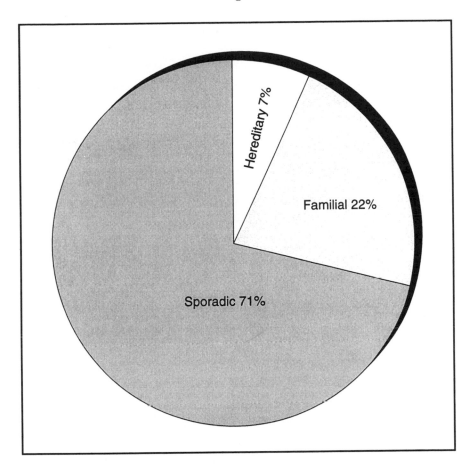

FIGURE 3

Percentages of New Breast Cancer Cases with a Genetic Component

Within such families, a sad chain of the disease is only too evident, passing from grandmother to mother, mother to daughter. Fortunately, the hereditary pattern of breast cancer is quite rare. Notice in Figure 3 just how few breast cancer cases have a positive family history (familial and hereditary).

Benign (Proliferative) Breast Disease

As we have already explained, the term *benign breast disease* can describe several related conditions. In general, however, any unusual growth or proliferation of breast cells is associated with some increased risk of malignancy.

Proliferative breast disease is the term often used to describe particularly dense breast tissue. This extra growth or proliferation of the breast's ducts and glands can be seen and measured on a woman's mammogram. An increased mammographic density pattern ("dense breasts" indicating increased rates of growth of breast cells) has been shown to carry a greater risk for future breast cancer.

Dr. John Wolfe was the first radiologist to demonstrate that breast-density patterns on a mammogram were a significant clue to a woman's later risk for a malignant breast tumor. The different patterns of mammogram densities are referred to as *Wolfe Grades*. Dr. Wolfe's studies have shown that the denser the breasts are in young women, the higher their risk for later malignant changes.

Age

The risk of developing a breast tumor increases with age. In a woman's early years, before the age of thirty, her chances of a malignant breast tumor are small. However, the risk quickly begins to rise as a woman reaches the age of menopause. The table shown on page 35 illustrates the relative likelihood of developing a breast tumor at any age.

CHANCES OF DEVELOPING BREAST CANCER
AT A GIVEN AGE

By age 25:	1 in 19,608
By age 30:	1 in 2,525
By age 35:	1 in 622
By age 40:	1 in 217
By age 45:	1 in 93
By age 50:	1 in 50
By age 55:	1 in 33
By age 60:	1 in 24
By age 65:	1 in 17
By age 70:	1 in 14
By age 75:	1 in 11
By age 80:	1 in 10
By age 85:	1 in 9
Over age 85:	1 in 8

Source: Surveillance, Epidemiology, and End Results (SEER) Program of the National Cancer Institute

Height

The discovery of a link between a woman's height and her risk for breast cancer may seem unusual. Nevertheless, several studies have confirmed the observation that the taller women in any given country have a greater risk. It has been suggested that taller stature simply reflects better nourishment as a child, or perhaps as a teenager. The breasts are thought to be more vulnerable to dietary influences at these early stages in their development. It is possible that higher caloric intake at relatively early ages affects stature as well as malignant processes in the breasts later in life.

How tall is tall? you might ask. In coming to their conclusion, researchers generally compared the breast cancer rates of the tallest women in a population with those of the shortest women. There-fore, tall in this context usually means well above the average height of *most* women in a country. It is difficult to set an exact height at which stature becomes a danger to the breasts. We can only be certain that the *tallest* women in a given country carry a somewhat higher risk than do the shortest ones.

Environmental Risk Factors

Oral Contraceptives

A possible link between the use of oral contraceptives and the later development of a malignant breast tumor has been a concern to women and their physicians for at least three decades. In 1989, it was estimated over 60 *million women* were using this medication worldwide.

Dozens of international committees have met over the years to debate the facts surrounding this issue. Their efforts have been complicated by changes in the pharmaceutical composition of oral contraceptives themselves. The basic change involved a gradual reduction in the amount of estrogen a woman received each day. It has been difficult, therefore, to compare the health effects of the pill in succeeding generations. Early research into the cancer risks of oral contraceptives was also hampered by the fact that many women simply had not been using them long enough to detect a possible harmful effect.

Nevertheless, based on the evidence, many physicians have come to believe that the use of oral contraceptives for many years in-creases a woman's relative risk of breast cancer by a factor of about 1.5. Given the tens of millions of women using this medication worldwide, however, scientists would like to know whether some groups of women are more susceptible to this danger than others. It may be that women with benign breast disease or those with a positive family history of breast cancer face the greatest risk from use of oral contraceptives. Further research will help to clarify these issues.

It is important to remember that oral contraceptives have certain benefits, as well. For example, their long-term use protects women against cancers of the ovary and the uterus. We simply do not yet know whether these benefits outweigh the increased breast cancer risk for the majority of women.

Estrogen Replacement Therapy

Medical scientists have concluded that the use of estrogen (with or without added progesterone) for alleviating postmenopausal symptoms and dangers, such as hot flashes or bone loss, increases the possibility of developing a malignant breast tumor. The increased risk is similar to that of oral contraceptive use.

The extent of increased danger with hormone replacement therapy depends upon the length of time a woman uses estrogen. Studies suggest that risk is not significantly increased until approximately five years of use. After that time, the additional risk increases with each year a woman uses the medication. Women with a positive family history of breast cancer appear to be even more susceptible to the cancer-causing effects of hormone replacement therapy.

As with oral contraceptives, a woman and her physician need to take several factors into account when deciding for *or* against estrogen replacement therapy. For example, some women, for genetic or other reasons, are at very high risk for bone fracture and/or heart disease. The benefit to these women from postmenopausal estrogen would likely outweigh the additional risks of breast or uterine cancer.

Women also vary considerably in the severity of their postmenopausal symptoms. For those with debilitating symptoms, the use of estrogen would be considered a necessity rather than a choice. The potential risks and benefits of using this important medication must be carefully considered by each woman and her physician.

Alcohol

Alcohol consumption has also recently been found to present an added risk for breast cancer. The risk seems to increase with the more alcohol a woman regularly drinks. Some studies suggest that as little as one drink per day, *on a regular basis,* can double a woman's chances of developing the disease. This important link between alcohol intake and breast malignancy needs further study.

Radiation

Exposure of the breasts to dangerous amounts of radiation is no longer very likely to occur. Nevertheless, in the past, some women's breasts were exposed unnecessarily during certain medical procedures, such as radiation to treat chronic acne or to shrink the thyroid. The risk for breast cancer is increased under these conditions.

Pesticide Exposure

Medical scientists have recently established that the pesticide DDT, if present in high levels in a woman's body, can increase her danger of developing a malignant breast tumor. Research conducted by Dr. Paolo Toniolo, a cancer epidemiologist at New York University School of Medicine, and his colleagues at Mount Sinai Hospital in New York found that a woman faced nearly a four times greater risk when the *highest* levels of DDE (the major breakdown product of DDT) were present in her bloodstream. Dr. Toniolo's work was corroborated just this year by a group of Canadian scientists who reported that estrogen-sensitive tumors were clearly linked to DDT exposure. These studies underscore the importance of ongoing investigations of environmental substances that may add to a woman's breast cancer risk.

Lifestyle Risk Factors

Diet

Breast cancer risk can be affected by several aspects of a woman's diet, including the total number of calories she eats, the amount of saturated fat consumed, the total amount of fat calories, the amount and type of fiber eaten, and the amount of fresh fruits and vegetables eaten each day. Each of the above variables contributes to a woman's overall diet, and each of them has been targeted by scientists either as a potential contributor or a probable deterrent to the overall incidence of breast cancer worldwide. We will consider each of these variables in more detail in later chapters.

When comparing women with high levels of dietary fat (over 40 percent of daily calories derived from fat) with women with low levels of dietary fat (around 30 percent of daily calories from fat), an increase in relative risk of 1.1 to 1.5 has been detected. If women with only 20 percent fat calories are compared, the relative risk from dietary fat may be even greater still.

Lack of Exercise

Aerobic exercise is believed to reduce the risk of breast cancer. The value of exercise is most apparent when it is performed on a regular basis, which usually means for at least thirty minutes three times each week. An important study in this area was performed by Dr. Rose Frisch at Harvard's Center for Population Studies. Dr. Frisch's research team contacted 5,398 female college alumnae, half of whom were former college athletes and the rest nonathletes. The rate of breast malignancies among the former athletes was only half of that among the other group of women who didn't exercise during college. In addition, the risk of other tumors of the reproductive system (uterus, ovary, cervix, and vagina) was also reduced by 60 to 70 percent among the athletes.

Obesity

Obesity is recognized to be an overall health risk, and obese women are at greater risk for breast cancer. Doctors usually define obesity as a woman's weight being greater than 20 percent above the level recommended for her height and frame. The increased risk to the breasts, however, seems to be present only among older women, over fifty years of age. This fact may be related to the observation that fat cells produce the hormone estrogen. Before menopause, women's bodies can adjust to any extra estrogen produced by fat cells by reducing the estrogen normally formed by the ovaries. In older obese women, however, such compensation by the ovaries is no longer possible. Since estrogen continually seeps out of fat cells, the risk for breast cancer among postmenopausal overweight women is consequently higher.

While total weight is a factor for breast cancer, the distribution of body-fat stores may also be crucial. Two recent studies of the health effects of body-fat distribution patterns reported that fat distributed mostly in the upper body (from the waist up, or "apple-shaped" pattern) is far more dangerous than fat stored mostly in the lower body (such as the hips and buttocks, or "pear-shaped" pattern).

Risk-Reduction Strategies Apply to All Women

As you begin to assess your own breast cancer risk, it will become immediately apparent that some of these factors cannot be changed. Your age at menarche, your family history, your height, and your age at menopause—these matters are beyond a woman's control.

Fortunately, there are a number of risk factors that you *can* influence. First, you can limit your alcohol intake. Second, you can maintain an active exercise program. Third, and most important, you can eat a breast-healthy diet. Our goal is to encourage you to make these changes in your diet and lifestyle today. Our message is that *every woman*, regardless of her individual history, can benefit to some extent from a program of breast cancer risk reduction.

The Cornerstone of Risk Reduction: A Breast-Healthy Diet

In 1981, two British scientists, Sir Richard Doll and his colleague Richard Peto, published an article titled, "The causes of cancer: quantitative estimates of avoidable risks of cancer in the United States today." In this important paper, quoted countless times by other scientists over the years, Doll and Peto provided strong evidence that *35 to 70 percent of all cancers* could potentially be prevented by a healthy diet! More than a decade later, as Professor Doll recently pointed out, the accumulating scientific evidence continues to support this link.

This strong relationship between food and cancer risk has led to the U.S. government recommendations found in the Five-a-Day for Better Health program. Scientists worldwide are coming to recognize the power of a healthy diet and lifestyle to reduce our risk from breast cancer and other chronic illnesses.

A risk-reduction program can be adopted by women of all ages. In younger women, such a strategy may prevent a tumor from forming or from becoming fully established. In older women, this approach may help to slow the growth and development of tumor cells already present.

However, the best way to fully understand the importance of diet in the development of breast cancer is by comparing disease rates in women living in different countries around the world. In the next chapter, we will show you how merely moving from one country to another can increase a woman's risk within just a few years.

CHAPTER THREE

WHO IN THE WORLD GETS BREAST CANCER?

Nutrition Influences Breast Disease Worldwide

Epidemiologists, the scientific sleuths of the medical community, have long been aware that women living in different parts of the world develop breast cancer at widely varying rates. In fact, in some countries the risk for this disease can be over *five to ten times* greater than in others.

In their efforts to understand these wide differences in risk, medical researchers have pored over the statistical data of millions of women around the world, carefully comparing the incidence and distribution of malignant breast tumors. For example, only 2 to 5 women per 100,000 die each year from this disease in such countries as Thailand and Sri Lanka. Yet breast cancer will claim the lives of 30 to 40 women per 100,000 in the United States and Great Britain. What can possibly account for such differences?

Scientists have struggled for decades to track down the elusive factors that account for such varying breast disease rates. The

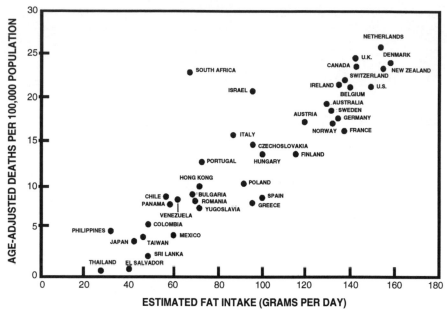

FIGURE 4

Worldwide Variations in Breast Cancer Deaths

United States, Great Britain, Holland, Canada, and New Zealand have much higher death rates from breast tumors, compared with such countries as Thailand, Japan, and the Philippines. Figure 4 shows the overall death rates from breast cancer in a number of countries around the world.

The percentage of animal fat in the diet has been pinpointed as a possible determining factor in the breast cancer rates of a country. Figure 4 indicates that breast cancer deaths around the world are much higher in countries where the fat consumption is also high. The study in which this figure originally appeared was published in 1968 by Dr. Kenneth Carroll and his colleagues. Although it has appeared numerous times in medical books and journals over the past twenty-five years, its value remains undiminished. The message it conveys is clear: *Nutrition influences the occurrence of breast disease around the world.*

Migration Studies: The West May Be Hazardous to Your Breasts

Shortly after World War II, scientists began to explore a different approach to understanding breast cancer differences around the world. Working with Japanese researchers in the late 1950s, scientists at the U.S. National Cancer Institute noted that Japanese women and their daughters who recently migrated to the United States developed a higher incidence of malignant breast tumors than women who did not emigrate.

Similar observations were made among descendants of Chinese women living in Hawaii. Many of the families of these women had already been living in Hawaii for two or three generations when these individuals were studied. Medical researchers were amazed to discover that their breast cancer rates were almost as high as those of the Caucasian women living in the same communities.

Data was also collected regarding the death rates from breast cancer of Polish women who had moved to the United States and Australia. Breast cancer in Poland, particularly among women living in farming communities, was relatively rare at the time. After migration, however, the breast cancer rates in these Polish women and their daughters quickly rose to the levels observed for American- and Australian-born Caucasian women.

In a follow-up study, it was found that Polish-born women who had moved to England and Wales also lost the "protection" against breast cancer they had previously enjoyed in Poland prior to their move. This second Polish study was particularly important, since it suggested how quickly changes can be seen in breast cancer rates as different dietary and lifestyle habits are adopted.

Other migration studies conducted on European women have also revealed the same remarkable results, as seen with Italian families emigrating to Australia. Shortly after arriving, these immigrants changed their traditional eating habits, due to the easy availability of meat and dairy products in Australia. In Italy, many of these families would have eaten traditional diets of pasta, fish, fruits and vegetables, and low-fat bread. Within one generation, breast cancer rates among these immigrants approached levels comparable to women born of European ancestry and raised in Australia.

In the 1990s, we continue to witness the crucial interaction of diet, geography, and breast cancer. Dr. Lenore Kohlmeier, head of the Department of Epidemiology of Health Risks at the German Federal Health Office in Berlin, has written that women living in former East Germany have lower breast cancer rates than their West German counterparts. Dr. Kohlmeier has proposed this may be due to the higher amount of cabbage and other vegetables consumed in the simpler diets of East German women.

"How Do International Breast Cancer Studies Apply to Me?"

Two important ideas emerge from studies of cancer in women who emigrate to other countries. First, the findings strongly indicate that *breast cancer rates are changeable.* The fact that a woman's chances of developing a breast malignancy may rise as soon as she moves to another country and abandons her former eating habits suggests the opposite may also be true. If women adopt diets closer to those of nontechnological, or "traditional," cultures, they could markedly reduce their own risk of breast cancer.

Second, studies of cancer rates in female immigrants demonstrate that the effects of diet are usually strongest in their daughters' generation. Dietary changes are apparently most important when made *early* in a woman's life, possibly even during late childhood, before a girl's first menstrual cycle.

Scientists recognize that positive changes made in the adolescent years protect the breasts while they are still developing. Such early changes in a young woman's life are believed to reduce the onset, or *initiation*, of DNA damage to the breasts. However, even for older women, there are important benefits from a change in dietary habits and lifestyle. In these women, positive dietary changes may slow the growth, or *promotion*, of a breast malignancy.

A major goal of breast cancer scientists, therefore, is to identify the specific aspects of diet and the critical differences in lifestyle responsible for the amazing variations observed in breast cancer rates worldwide. Which factors, researchers ask, matter most in the lives of Japanese and Thai women who still follow a traditional lifestyle and diet? Which factors in the traditional Polish, Italian, or East German lifestyle and cuisine protected women so well prior to their emigration and assimilation into another culture? How do these lifestyles and dietary choices differ from those of the average American woman?

Components of a Traditional Diet and Lifestyle

Several cultural factors have an impact on the risk of developing breast cancer. When researchers studied the lives of women in various traditional agricultural societies, they noticed a consistent pattern associated with lower breast cancer rates.

DIET AND LIFESTYLE FACTORS LINKED TO CANCER PROTECTION IN TRADITIONAL CULTURES

DIETARY	LIFESTYLE
Lower total dietary fat calories	Lower total body weight
Lower total calorie intake	More daily exercise
More legumes, whole grains	Earlier first childbirth
More fruits and vegetables	Larger numbers of children
Lower intake of saturated fats	Later onset of menstruation

The protective aspects of lifestyle have been most clearly seen in studies of women living in Asian countries, such as Japan and China. In these societies, women are generally slimmer than their Western counterparts. Studies as early as the 1950s by Japanese researchers indicated that Asian women usually had their first menstrual period significantly later in life (between fifteen and seventeen years of age) than most American girls (as early as eleven to twelve years of age). Even in the 1990s, the situation has changed little in China. Scientists at the Tianjin Cancer Institute continue to observe the relatively late onset of menarche among Chinese girls, as well as the protective influence this ultimately has on breast cancer.

Women living in traditional agricultural societies often marry earlier in life. They not only give birth to more children but they begin to have those children at a younger age. They are more likely to breast-feed their infants and continue to do so for longer periods of time for each child than American mothers.

Also, with fewer laborsaving devices, Asian women in a traditional setting tend to get more exercise than women in this country. Women in agrarian cultures usually eat far more vegetables, whole grains, legumes, and fruits, and relatively little meat, compared with American women. These foods contain large amounts of different types of dietary fiber. In addition, they contain a remarkable array of protective plant chemicals.

Diets high in vegetables also contain less saturated fat. Traditional eating habits favor a diet low in saturated fat, low in calories from fats, and low in total calories. Moreover, the actual fat in such diets is usually of the safer monounsaturated or polyunsaturated type (for example, olive oil, peanut oil, or omega-3 fish oils). These oils substitute for the more dangerous saturated fats common in Western diets.

Japan: A Living Laboratory for Breast Cancer Research

In order to understand how dietary changes can affect breast cancer rates over time, we must study a country where the dietary pattern is slowly beginning to resemble our own. When medical scientists first examined the dietary habits of Japanese women before World War II, they found most women followed a pattern similar to other traditional societies. More importantly, they observed the blessing of a low rate of breast cancer among these women. In the postwar years, however, sweeping changes took place in Japanese society. Families became smaller and an urban lifestyle largely replaced the rural lifestyle for three out of four Japanese. There was also a noticeable rise in the employment status of women, especially among younger women.

With the influx of these Western influences has come an enormous change in the eating habits of the country, as documented by the Japanese National Nutrition Survey. This survey, conducted routinely by the Japanese Ministry of Health and Welfare in November every year since 1945, interviews about twenty thousand persons in approximately seven thousand households randomly selected throughout Japan. The National Nutrition Survey shows that the Japanese have not only enthusiastically embraced jeans, jogging shoes, and rock music; they have also adopted American tastes in food.

This fundamental change in the Japanese cuisine is most evident in meat consumption. Japan is now a major importer of American beef products, consistently buying more than half of all U.S. beef exports. In 1991 alone, according to the U.S. Meat Export Federation in Denver, the Japanese purchased over $1.2 billion in beef products.

SELECTED CHANGES IN EATING HABITS IN JAPAN FROM 1960 TO 1980

Average Yearly Consumption of Various Food Items (per person in kilograms)

YEAR	RICE	VEGETABLES	MEAT	EGGS	MILK PRODUCTS
1960	114.9	100.0	5.0	6.3	22.3
1965	111.7	109.6	9.2	11.6	37.4
1970	95.1	115.6	13.4	14.8	50.1
1975	88.1	111.3	17.9	14.0	53.3
1980	78.9	112.2	22.4	14.6	62.2

Source: Japanese National Nutrition Survey

As the table shows, the Japanese demand for meat, eggs, and milk products has skyrocketed. Rice consumption, the traditional staple of Japanese diets, declined nearly 40 percent during this same period. While the demand for high-fat foods has increased dramatically in Japan, the consumption of vegetables has hardly changed at all.

Japanese rice farmers have watched as more and more of their cropland has been turned over to raising cattle. "Japanese rice farming is like a person on a bed barely surviving with an oxygen mask," noted a farmer in a recent interview. The number of farm households in Japan has steadily decreased from over 6 million to only 3.8 million, and livestock has surpassed rice as the nation's number-one agricultural product. The Japanese beef industry is famous for its *wagyu,* or Kobe, beef. This product comes from massaged and pampered cattle fed a rich diet of soybeans, grains, and beer—all designed to raise the meat's fat content to over twenty-six grams per four-ounce serving.

While few Japanese families can afford a Kobe steak, other dietary changes have taken place in Japan that are not all for the better. Within the past generation, for example, fast-food restaurants have popped up like mushrooms in Japanese cities. According to the McDonald's Corporation, 604 of their fast-food restaurants were present in Japan in 1987, climbing to a whopping 865 by 1991—the highest number of any country in the world, except the United States. Pepsico, Inc., owners of Pizza Hut, Kentucky Fried Chicken, and Taco Bell, has also successfully targeted the Japanese market, according to their 1991 annual financial report.

In addition, ice cream has become a great favorite among the Japanese. Grand Met, the huge international company behind the Burger King chain, as well as the manufacturer of one of the richest ice creams in the world, Häagen-Dazs, states in its 1991 annual report, "In the Far East, Häagen-Dazs is the number one superpremium ice cream in *Japan* through a joint venture that controls product manufacture and distribution, including 81 retail shops." The dietary fat content in a single serving (four ounces) of these Häagen-Dazs products is around twenty grams—or more than the entire daily fat consumption for many of these Japanese under a more traditional diet!

It was only a matter of time before the health effects of these altered dietary patterns in Japan would be noticed. By the early 1970s, medical researchers began to observe disturbing changes in the health of Japanese women. The death rate from breast cancer was increasing.

In 1977, Dr. Takeshi Hirayama, a prominent medical scientist, warned about the dangerous influence of diet in the growth of breast tumors among Japanese women. He singled out the harmful role of dietary fat, "the intake of which is increasing rapidly." Dr. Hirayama added, "This was shown clearly by our ongoing cancer population-based prospective studies in Japan. A significantly higher standardized mortality ratio of breast cancer *in women with a habit of daily meat intake* was observed."

It is important to remember these changes took place in Japan so rapidly after World War II that researchers had difficulty in properly assessing the mechanisms linking diet and breast cancer. By the time biochemical and hormonal studies were performed in the 1980s, it was difficult to find Japanese women who still followed a purely traditional lifestyle.

The pattern emerging from all of these studies is clear: Dietary choices influence breast cancer rates worldwide. To put this conclusion in different terms, we can say that a woman's dietary choices affect her risk. This holds true whether she lives in a "protective" society or moves to a "high risk" society.

These careful observations of whole populations at risk around the world reveal *how* diet can work to protect you (and your family) against the threat of breast disease. But what is it, specifically, about a woman's diet that places her at such varying degrees of risk? *Why* do such recommendations as the Five-a-Day program work, and which five vegetables would be helpful for breast cancer? We still have not examined whether it is simply the amount of animal fat a woman consumes each day, as suggested by Dr. Hirayama, that determines her risk. Is some other dietary component also involved?

A number of research studies have attempted to answer these vital questions. The accumulated results suggest that we must move beyond the assumption that dietary fat is the *sole* culprit in the diet-breast cancer link. Rather, we need to understand how all of the components of a healthy diet play a role in this disease.

THE DIETARY FAT/BREAST CANCER DEBATE

A wealth of scientific evidence supports the position that a woman's dietary choices can influence her overall risk for breast cancer. Yet even with all of the data amassed by researchers on this subject, our understanding of the diet-breast cancer puzzle is still incomplete.

Most breast cancer physicians and researchers have usually looked to *excessive fat calories* as the *primary* troublemaker in our diets. It is easy to understand why fat has been singled out: At present, fat makes up over 40 *percent* of the total daily calories eaten by many women.

Laboratory studies of dietary fat and breast tumors in animals have provided strong supporting evidence for the dangerous role of fat in the development of breast cancer. Studies of the association between dietary fat and breast cancer in humans, however, have been difficult to perform and to interpret. This uncertainty has resulted in an open debate about the role of dietary fat as a risk factor, not only for breast cancer but for other malignancies, as well.

Animal Studies of Dietary Fat and Breast Tumors

The connection between a high-fat diet and breast cancer has been extensively researched for over half of this century. In 1942, Professor Albert Tannenbaum reported that female mice fed a diet high in fat calories had an increased rate of malignant breast tumors. Since then, literally thousands of additional research studies have been carried out to clarify this link. While breast tumors in experimental animals differ in important ways from those in women, laboratory studies of dietary fat have clearly shed light upon the factors affecting the relationship of fat consumption and human breast cancer risk.

Researchers have come to realize that the dangerous effect of fat in the diet is linked to *the total amount of calories* an experimental animal consumes. When there is no limitation on the number of calories available to an animal, then high amounts of dietary fat invariably cause a great deal of damage to its breasts. When researchers limit the amount of calories the animal is able to eat each day, however, the cancerous effect of fat is greatly reduced.

Research scientists have also discovered that different types of fat vary in their ability to promote the growth of animal tumors. Saturated fats, such as lard, beef tallow, and palm and coconut oils, were usually more dangerous than unsaturated vegetable oils. The safest were the omega-3 unsaturated oils, or the so-called fish oils, which are also found in plants in a form called linolenic acid.

Other laboratory studies have shown that breast tumors in animals are more likely to spread throughout the body, or metastasize, when dietary fat calories are higher. All of these results suggest similar effects may occur in women eating fat-rich foods.

Dietary Fat and Breast Cancer in Women

The evidence from animal studies, as well as the epidemiological observations we previously discussed, led many researchers to believe it would be an open-and-shut case to implicate fat as the major culprit for breast cancer risk in women. However, proving their case has not been so simple.

On one side of the debate are those who maintain that a high intake of dietary fat is a major driving force behind elevated breast cancer rates in women. Support for this position was recently offered by a team of international scientists led by Dr. Geoffrey Howe. This group combined the results from twelve individual studies of diet and breast cancer risk involving over 10,500 women. They reported a significantly increased risk for breast cancer in older women who had higher levels of saturated-fat intake. The researchers concluded about 16 percent of breast cancers in younger women, and up to 24 percent in older women, might be prevented by substantially lowering their dietary fat.

If they are correct, a relatively simple dietary change could translate into tens of thousands of American women each year who would not have to hear the diagnosis, "You have breast cancer."

Dr. Walter Willett and his associates at the Harvard Medical School, however, take a different stand. They believe dietary fat is not the villain in breast cancer. Their conclusion is based upon an ongoing analysis of breast cancer rates among more than 89,000 female nurses whom they have been following for over eight years (called the Nurses' Health Study). Their latest results were published in October 1992 in the *Journal of the American Medical Association.*

Dr. Willett's team did not observe any protective effect on breast cancer rates due to lower fat intake among these nurses, although they did note that lower-fat diets seemed to lower the risks of heart disease and colon cancer. Based upon these findings, Dr. Willett concluded, "There is no suggestion of an association [between fat calories and breast cancer] no matter what type of fat you consider." Results from this major study have continued to fuel the ongoing dietary fat/breast cancer debate.

Although Dr. Willett's results would lead some to believe that dietary fat plays little, if any, role in breast cancer rates, many cancer experts have seriously questioned this conclusion. The differences in levels of fat consumption among the women in the

Nurses' Health Study are relatively small, for example, suggesting that few differences in breast cancer rates could ever be found in this group of nurses.

A large proportion of the women in the Nurses' Health Study were already eating a Western diet, high in fat calories, during the eight years of their follow-up. They were never taught how they might specifically improve their diets by lowering the fat. As a result, very few of the participants actually ate a *very low-fat diet*. Many scientists think that a low-fat diet contributes to breast health *only* when a woman limits fat to 20 percent or less of her daily calories. Consequently, critics insist that these women would first have to be taught how to recognize and then eat a truly low-fat diet in order for the study to be meaningful.

Moreover, the dietary questionnaire used by Dr. Willett's team has been judged by many nutritionists to be inaccurate in determining the precise amount of fat eaten each day. In the Nurses' Health Study, women were asked on a given day to recall what foods they had eaten, on average, over the past two years. They completed a similar questionnaire on four separate occasions during the eight-year study. Most of us would be unable to remember correctly what we ate over the past two weeks, let alone over the past two years.

Food preparation was an additional factor not taken fully into account in this dietary questionnaire. For example, was the chicken they ate baked, fried, steamed, or grilled? Was it served with or without skin, with or without a sauce? Each of these choices can greatly affect a meal's fat content.

In an editorial accompanying the 1992 report of the Nurses' Health Study, Dr. Howe reminds us that at least three other recent research projects, similar in design to Dr. Willett's study, had found that higher amounts of dietary fat increased breast cancer risk. Thus, the debate among researchers goes on.

Which group of experts is right and which is wrong? And where does this leave women who are trying to sort out the opposing viewpoints? Barbara Kronman, codirector of SHARE, a self-help advocacy group for women with breast cancer, expressed the reaction of many women to the debate over the Nurses' Health Study: "I think women will be disappointed and not really believe it. This is one of the few areas in which we can feel some control over our lives. If this gets taken away from us, we are left with a very fatalistic approach."

There is a simple explanation why scientific studies of fat and breast cancer in women are so controversial. It is, in fact, quite difficult to know *exactly* what a woman eats during the course of her life and just how much fat is actually in her diet. Researchers have often observed that people inaccurately report what they are eating.

In two separate detailed studies, for example, groups of men and women were first carefully taught how to fill out a detailed food diary. Using independent biochemical methods to check the accuracy of their food records, scientists found that many people underestimated their intake by at least seven hundred to one thousand calories each day. The troubling conclusion is that by using only surveys and questionnaires, we may never be able to know for sure how much fat is in a woman's diet.

A much better research approach would be to first *teach women how to prepare and follow a low-fat diet*. Breast cancer rates could then be compared over time between these women and another group of women who were not specifically taught how to follow such a diet. This "prospective" approach was incorporated into the design of the Women's Health Trial.

The Women's Health Trial: Teaching Women to Eat Right

By the mid-1980s, it was clear that a different approach was needed to determine whether reducing fat in the diet would, in fact, protect women's breasts. This concern led to an ambitious research effort termed the Women's Health Trial, or WHT, spearheaded by Dr. Maureen M. Henderson of the Fred Hutchinson Cancer Research Center in Seattle.

Dr. Henderson and her colleagues had come to believe that a low-fat eating trial was *the only way* to answer definitively the dietary fat/breast cancer debate. As she put it, "No other research design can give a *direct* answer to a question about the impact of a dietary change."

The WHT was therefore planned as a nationwide randomized study to determine specifically whether a low-fat diet would reduce the risk of breast cancer. The researchers originally estimated it would be necessary to follow 32,000 women from twelve different large U.S. cities, ages forty-five to sixty-nine years, for at least ten years in order to see a drop of 17 percent in breast malignancies. The cost for such a study would be around $100 million.

From the outset, the WHT researchers needed to answer two simple questions. First, could large numbers of women be successfully taught to change their dietary habits? And second, would women really be able to *maintain* healthy dietary changes over a long period of time?

In order to settle the first issue—whether a large group of women could learn to eat a diet low in fat calories—WHT researchers enrolled 303 women in Seattle, Cincinnati, and Houston into a preliminary program known as the Vanguard Study. In this pilot study, three out of five women participants were randomly placed in an intervention group and given extensive attention from a nutritionist acting as educator and counselor. Groups of eight to fifteen women met weekly for the first two months to discuss diet plans, then biweekly for one month, and monthly for the rest of the two-year study. Each woman had two individual sessions with the nutritionist, as well. The control group included the other two of the five women randomly selected. These women were seen every six months for a dietary assessment but were not given any specific advice about dietary fat modifications. All of the participants were followed for at least two years.

The results of the WHT Vanguard Trial were startling in their success. First of all, women in the intervention group readily accepted the changes needed to reduce fat calories in their diets. They did such things as cutting back on red meat, sampling new recipes, switching from whole-fat to low-fat or nonfat dairy products, using less cream or cheese sauces with vegetables, and eating more fruit.

By making these few simple modifications, they reduced the amount of fat in their diets to around 22 to 25 percent of calories, down from the nearly 40 percent typical of most American women.

Indeed, women in the intervention group were largely successful because they chose manufactured foods that were already low in fat and they modified commonly used foods and recipes, making them lower in fat. The researchers were careful not to forbid the women to eat any specific food. Instead, participants were taught how to keep track of the amount of fat they ate each day and how to make simple choices and substitutions to lower the fat whenever possible. The overall goal was to interfere as little as possible with a woman's normal dietary habits.

WHT scientists were excited to find that the intervention group in the Vanguard Study accomplished four other important goals without realizing it. First, they ate about four hundred fewer calories each day compared with the control group of women. This fact alone would very likely have a beneficial health effect. Second, the changes in their diets resulted in a lowering of blood-cholesterol levels by an average of fifteen points. Third, it was observed that their husbands began to eat a lower-fat diet, as well. This benefit for the men probably occurred merely as a result of living in the same household as a woman in the intervention group.

The fourth and most important result was a *reduction in estrogen hormones* in women eating the low-fat diets. This provocative finding was the clearest indication that dietary improvement is likely to be protective to the breasts.

Obviously, women can be taught in large numbers to eat a healthier diet. But would they continue to do so years later? The answer to this was also a clear *yes*. Women in the intervention group maintained the percentage of calories from fat at a level around 20 to 25 percent for the full two years of the study. There was very little return to the old eating habits.

After the Vanguard Study was completed, nearly all of the women were interviewed again, at least one year after their last contact with the nutrition team. Researchers discovered that most women who had been taught to eat a low-fat diet continued to eat that way.

The Women's Health Trial also discovered that women who limited their fat intake soon lost their taste for fatty foods. Within six months, many of the participants in this program actually found such fatty foods distasteful.

Despite the success of the pilot-phase Vanguard Study, however, a full fifteen-year, $107 million revised Women's Health Trial, scheduled to begin in 1991, was canceled at the last moment by the scientific advisory board of the National Cancer Institute. Critics of the WHT still insist such large-scale dietary trials are impossible to conduct properly. It was one thing to follow 303 women closely over two years, they argue—but 24,000 to 32,000 women over fifteen years?

It does not appear likely that the Women's Health Trial will be conducted in the United States in the near future. Instead, a variation of the WHT, called the Women's Health Initiative, was funded under the leadership of Dr. Bernadine Healy, former Director of the National Institutes of Health. This research initiative is expected to cost over $500 million by the time it is completed in ten years. The purpose of the Women's Health Initiative is to investigate the relationship of diet to such diseases as breast cancer, osteoporosis, and heart disease in women.

Unfortunately, the focus of the Women's Health Initiative is no longer only *dietary fat and breast cancer*. Many breast cancer researchers fear this new initiative is overambitious and much too complicated. Moreover, critics do not believe that it will settle the critical issues in the dietary fat/breast cancer debate.

Even as we await the outcome of the Women's Health Initiative over the next decade, the evidence of the Vanguard phase of the WHT is clear: *Women can make lasting changes in their diets now.*

A Low-Fat Diet Isn't Enough

If fat alone cannot explain rising breast cancer rates, then what does? Even though a link between diet and breast cancer is definitely at work, fat calories alone do not account for much of the differences

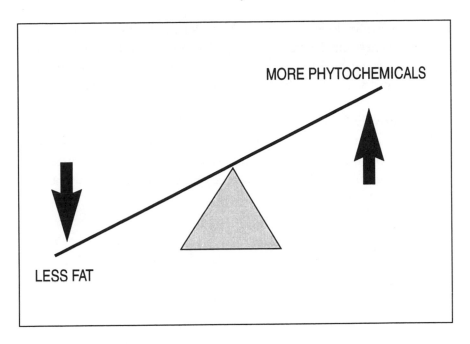

FIGURE 5

Either Lowering Fat or Increasing Fruits and Vegetables
Will Have a Similar Effect on Your Diet

among women at risk. Medical research suggests that a breast-healthy diet involves several factors *other than fat.*

As Figure 5 shows, a low-fat diet will almost always be abundant in plant products: fruits, vegetables, and grains. This simple relationship is extremely important, since it shifts the focus away from fat as the main culprit in breast cancer rates. The figure also brings home the fact it is possible to approach food with two entirely different attitudes.

We believe that the *missing piece of the breast cancer puzzle* involves the remarkable properties of fruits, vegetables, and grains in our diets. Medical scientists are just beginning to understand the enormous complexity of plant foods and the unusual phytochemical substances they contain.

Rather than looking at a healthy diet as an *absence*, or giving up, of something (such as the rich taste of fat calories), we can view the same healthy diet as the *presence* of breast-healthy fruits, grains, and vegetables, and their powerful phytochemical constituents.

By actively seeking to fit the suggested five to nine servings of fresh fruits and vegetables into our daily lives, we will also be eating a low-fat diet. The potential role of these plant substances in promoting our good health will be explored in the next chapter.

CHAPTER FIVE ──────────────────────────

BEYOND FAT:
THE PROTECTIVE EFFECTS OF
FRUITS AND VEGETABLES

If a cancerous ulcer appears on the breasts,
apply crushed cabbage leaf and it will make it well.
—Cato the Elder, 150 B.C.

This prescription by Cato the Elder, an ancient Roman statesman, might seem more an example of ancient quackery than ancient wisdom. Such a remedy would probably strike most people these days as strange, if not comical. Yet Cato's recommendation recalls a past in which the medicinal powers of plants were much more widely recognized and appreciated than they generally are now.

Various herbs and plants were honored in the ancient world for their curative properties. Even the humble cabbage was noted for its medicinal powers. As Cato wrote long ago, "It will purge wounds full of pus, and cancers, and make them well when no other treatment can accomplish it." While we would not prescribe crushed cabbage leaf today as a treatment for breast cancer, the presence of cancer-fighting phytochemicals in cruciferous vegetables such as cabbage is a proven fact.

It is ironic that medical science is finally corroborating some of the practical discoveries of ancient and traditional medicine. The unique health-promoting value of a simple lifestyle that includes a diet abundant in fresh fruits, vegetables, and grains is finally gaining the recognition it deserves.

Low Fat Equals High Phytochemicals

The beneficial effects of plant-based foods certainly should come as no surprise. The amounts of fruits and vegetables in a person's diet usually run in *opposite* proportion to the grams of fat eaten each day. Fat calories currently satisfy, on average, nearly 40 percent of our daily energy needs. Something has had to give way to make room for this increase in fat calories over the years—and it was the fresh fruits, vegetables, and whole grains that were squeezed out of the picture.

In the following table, compare the nutritional properties of foods made predominantly from plants with those foods based on animal fat and proteins.

COMPARISON OF PLANT-BASED VERSUS HIGH-FAT FOODS

FOODS RICH IN FRUITS, VEGETABLES, GRAINS	FOODS RICH IN ANIMAL FATS
Very low calorie density	High calorie density
Abundant in vitamins C and B complex	Low in water-soluble vitamins
High in natural fiber, complex carbohydrates	Low in fiber and carbohydrates
Abundant in natural phytochemicals	Absent in phytochemicals
Abundant amounts of antioxidants	Produce lipid peroxides that destroy antioxidants

This simple side-by-side comparison clearly shows the enormous potential health benefits from a diet built around vegetables, whole grains, and fruits, as opposed to one that derives its calories largely from oils and fatty meats. A diet rich in fruits and vegetables will almost always be low in fat.

A breast-healthy diet, then, involves far more than simply removing the fat from your menu. It requires a disciplined effort to replace those fat calories with plant-based foods. A bountiful supply of vitamins, minerals, fibers, and a host of unique chemicals supplied by the plants themselves is present in these foods.

Protection Against Cancer from Fruits and Vegetables

Two extensive surveys of the cancer-preventive effects of plant foods were published in 1991 and 1992. These studies left no doubt whatsoever about the power of plant-based foods to affect our good health. Drs. John Potter and Karen Steinmetz, scientists at the University of Minnesota, began their research on this topic by considering the historical association between eating fruits and vegetables and certain health benefits. They cited the Roman naturalist Pliny, who wrote that the consumption of cabbage was believed to cure over eighty-seven different illnesses, while eating onions was said to cure twenty-eight diseases. In fact, they explained that all sorts of vegetables have been used over thousands of years for their medicinal properties, including celery, cucumber, endive, parsley, peas, and many others.

The scientists then carefully reviewed over 130 modern scientific studies to determine whether the historical associations between vegetables and fruits and cancer had any basis in fact. Their findings were striking: *Higher consumption of fruits and vegetables was consistently associated with a much lower risk of cancer at most sites of the body.*

In the case of lung cancer, for example, all of the research studies examined by Potter and Steinmetz showed *a lower risk* among people eating the greatest amounts of fruits and vegetables. We have summarized some of their remarkable findings about the protective effects of a high fruit/vegetable diet in the following table.

NUMBER OF RESEARCH STUDIES SHOWING A CANCER-PREVENTING EFFECT OF A HIGH FRUIT AND VEGETABLE DIET

Lung cancer	8 of 8 studies
Colorectal cancers	18 of 23 studies
Esophageal cancer	10 of 11 studies
Larynx cancer	4 of 4 studies
Oral cancer	6 of 8 studies
Stomach cancer	15 of 17 studies
Pancreatic cancer	7 of 7 studies
Bladder cancer	3 of 3 studies
Breast cancer	3 of 5 studies
Uterine cancer	2 of 2 studies

Evidence was also found for the protective effect of diets high in fruits and vegetables against hormone-related cancers in women. Three out of five studies showed lower breast cancer rates linked to higher consumption of fruits and vegetables. Two studies of uterine cancer found that rates were reduced by 60 to 70 percent among women eating the greatest amounts of these types of foods.

The second research study to examine the relationship between consumption of fruits and vegetables and protection against cancer was performed by scientists at the National Cancer Institute and the University of California at Berkeley, led by Dr. Gladys Block. This review examined nearly two hundred published scientific reports. Again the results were striking. In nearly all organs of the body, the scientists found *cancer rates were cut by half or more* in those people who ate the most fresh fruits and vegetables.

In Dr. Block's findings, the protective effects of a high vegetable/ fruit diet also extended specifically to breast cancer. Although this disease has always been difficult to study because of the multiple risk factors involved, the NCI team nevertheless reported that a fruit and vegetable–based diet was protective against breast cancer.

The researchers were able to show that the benefits of fruits and vegetables were independent of those obtained by eating less fat calories. In fact, it was the combination of lowered fat *and* increased plant-food consumption that, added together, shielded women from the development of malignant breast tumors. The conclusions of both studies are clear: *A diet high in fruits and vegetables can reduce your overall cancer risk, and this protective umbrella extends to breast cancer, as well.*

Phytochemicals Are a Plant's Natural Pharmacy

What can explain the impressive properties of fruits and vegetables in prevention of human cancers? The answer is to be found within the plant itself. The components that make up a fruit or vegetable are more than a combination of water, starch, and fiber. Fruits, whole grains, and vegetables also contain a complex and amazing assortment of vitamins, minerals, and other remarkable chemicals found only in plants.

Most of these plant substances are vitally important if we are to maintain good health. The vast majority of these chemicals cannot be manufactured in our own bodies. Instead, we must rely upon eating a wide variety of plant-based foods to get a plentiful supply.

For example, you may have heard of the disease called scurvy. It used to be fairly common, especially among sailors up until the end of the eighteenth century. During long sea voyages, the men rarely ate fresh fruits and vegetables, surviving instead on salted beef and dry biscuits. As a result, any wound these men received healed poorly; their gums and mouths became sore and their teeth often loosened. The sailors would lose their appetite and develop anemia. However, in 1795, the Royal Navy recognized simply stocking their ships with fresh limes would completely alleviate the problem. To this day, British sailors are sometimes called limeys.

How did plants develop many of their amazing phytochemicals? Plants very gradually evolved these unique substances to protect themselves from the risk of being overeaten, whether by insects, grazing animals, or humans. These chemical agents usually functioned in some way to protect the plant, whether by providing a bitter taste to discourage animals from eating them or by acting as an antibiotic chemical to prevent attack by fungi or bacteria.

As we humans satisfied our nutritional needs by eating plants, we lost our own ability to produce some of the vitamins and amino acids they contain. In addition, the human body also developed the ability to make good use of many other phytochemicals in those plants. Several plant foods, particularly the leafy green vegetables, provide us with necessary vitamin A. But vitamin A is only a single member of a huge family of phytochemicals called *carotenoids*. One carotenoid frequently discussed in the media is beta-carotene, which is a building block for vitamin A. Yet there are at least *five hundred other carotenoids* in plants, such as lutein in parsley and spinach, lycopene in tomatoes, and many, many more.

The carotenoids in plant foods help our cells to trap active oxygen molecules. In this way, they function as *anti*oxidants and help to prevent the damaging effects of activated oxygen molecules on our tissues' DNA.

Some carotenoids may actually function just like vitamin A in reversing cancerous changes in cells. We will speak about how vitamin A may protect the breasts in a later chapter. Though we still understand relatively little about this huge family of remarkable phytochemicals, one thing is certain: The more vegetables we eat, the more of these substances our bodies have available to use to fight disease.

Dr. Christopher Beecher at the University of Illinois has worked for the past several years to create a computerized data base of the different phytochemicals contained in several common plant foods.

The astounding fact is most plants contain literally *hundreds* of chemicals. Some are simple and well known, like potassium, amino acids, and sugars, while others are complex and little known. As one can see in the following list, a single carrot or a serving of broccoli is full of an amazing number of phytochemicals.

EXAMPLES OF UNUSUAL PHYTOCHEMICALS IN COMMON VEGETABLES

CARROTS	BROCCOLI
Aesculetin	p-Hydroxybenzoic acid
Apigenin	Caffeic acid
Arachidonic acid	Beta-carotene
p-Hydroxybenzoic acid	Chlorogenic acid
Caffeic acid	Chlorophyll
Beta-carotene	Cinnamic acid
Chlorogenic acid	p-Coumaric acid
Chlorophyll	24-Methyl-cycloartanol
Chrysin	Ferulic acid
Cinnamic acid	trans-Ferulic acid
p-Coumaric acid	Glucobrassicin
Eugenol	Indole-3-carbinol
Ferulic acid	Indole-3-acetonitrile
Geraniol	3,3'-Diindolylmethane
Beta-ionone	Ascorbigen
Kaempherol	Kaempherol
Limonene	Linolenic acid
Linalool	Oleic acid
Linolenic acid	Phytic acid
Luteolin	Quercetin
Methionine	Rutin
Myristicin	Salicylic acid
Oleic acid	Sinapic acid
Alpha-pinene	Sinigrin
Psoralen	Squalene

5-Methoxypsoralen	Stigmasterol
Quercetin	Allyl-isothiocyanate
Quercitrin	Phenylethyl-isothiocyanate
Scopoletin	Vanillic acid
Beta-sitosterol	Ascorbic acid
Stigmasterol	Dithiolthione
Umbelliferone	Sulforaphane
Vanillic acid	

Were you surprised by the length of these lists? How many of these exotic-sounding chemicals did you recognize? And these are only some of the chemical compounds found in just two common vegetables. What, then, are the other leading plant contenders with pharmaceutical-like properties?

Garlic alone may provide us with over two hundred different, unusual chemicals capable of safeguarding us against a wide array of human diseases. Many of these chemical compounds contain sulfur; they seem to act *by increasing the production of protective enzymes in our bodies.* Garlic does not have to be eaten raw to be effective. You can cook it and reap the same rewards. Also, you may already be familiar with the odorless forms of garlic available today, which appear to be as effective as cooked garlic, if not more so. In Germany and Japan, a high percentage of the population takes a daily garlic supplement to help protect their health.

Green tea is another example of a potential cancer-fighter in our diets. Green tea is unfamiliar to many Americans and may still sound a bit strange. The tea we normally drink is actually made from green tea leaves darkened by a fermentation process.

Green tea, however, is favored by millions of people living in Japan, China, and other parts of Asia. The Tea Council and the Tea Association of the U.S.A., Inc., have reported that some people in Asia drink up to twelve cups of this beverage each day. Green tea is rich in chemicals called polyphenols, which act by soaking up activated oxygen molecules in the body. These compounds also appear to aid the immune system, lower cholesterol levels, and protect against various forms of cancer.

Another group of plants with pharmaceutical-like properties is the parsley, or umbelliferous, family of vegetables. It includes parsley, carrots, fennel, celery, and such common herbs as caraway seed, dill, cumin, and coriander. These vegetables contain strange-sounding compounds called coumarins and phenolics, which act in numerous ways to promote health. They prevent the formation of harmful nitrosamines in our intestines and elevate the production of our body's protective enzymes.

These three families of vegetables and their unique phytochemical makeup represent only a small fraction of the compounds we *could be eating* on a daily basis. They serve to remind us of the enormous potential for fruits, grains, and vegetables as storehouses of natural substances aimed directly against cancer processes in our bodies. The table on page 72 summarizes much of what scientists currently understand about the cancer fighting phytochemicals available to all of us in the foods we could be eating.

A Guide to the Plant Foods Important in Human Nutrition

Human beings have been experimenting with plants through a slow process of trial and error extending over thousands of years. In more recent times, agricultural scientists have worked actively to create entirely new varieties of vegetables, grains, and fruits in order to maximize one property or another of a particular plant. Growers produce seedless grapes, sturdier tomatoes, sweeter carrots, green cauliflowers, and many more exotic varieties to come. Most of the plants we eat and take for granted today never actually existed as such in the wild but, instead, slowly evolved along with different methods of agriculture.

The table on pages 73–75 lists the most widely eaten vegetables, grains, and fruits in our diet. They are grouped, when possible, according to various families. As you study this table, ask yourself the following simple questions. Do you know what these vegetables

POTENTIAL CANCER FIGHTERS IN FOODS

PHYTOCHEMICAL	PROTECTIVE MECHANISM	FOOD SOURCES
Allyl sulfides	Increase activity of protective enzymes in the body	Garlic and onions
Carotenoids	Act as antioxidants and help cells to differentiate	Parsley, carrots, winter squash, sweet potatoes, kale, spinach, apricots
Polyphenols	Act as antioxidants, and reduce danger of nitrosamines	Green tea, carrots, broccoli, cucumbers, squash, mint, basil, citrus fruits
Bioflavonoids	Block receptor sites for some hormones and enzymes	Most fruits, vegetables
Isoflavones	Block estrogen receptor, block tumor blood vessels, inhibit other tumor enzymes	Soybeans and other legumes
Indoles	Induce protective enzymes, stimulate C-2 estrogen production	Cabbage, broccoli, and Brussels sprouts
Isothiocyanates	Induce protective enzymes	Mustard, horseradish, radishes
Limonoids	Induce protective enzymes	All citrus fruits
Linolenic acid	Regulates production of prostaglandins in cells	Many leafy vegetables, seeds, particularly flaxseed
Monoterpenes	Antioxidant properties, induce protective enzymes	Parsley family, squash, basil, eggplant, mint, citrus fruits, tomatoes
Plant sterols	Help cells remain differentiated (non-cancerous)	Broccoli, cabbage, soy, peppers, whole grains
Sulforaphane	Induces protective enzymes	Broccoli, other cabbage family vegetables
Vitamin E	Antioxidant	Wheat germ, oatmeal, peanuts, brown rice

This table has been reproduced by permission of *Eating Well* magazine.

and fruits look like? Could you find them in the produce section of your food market if you wanted to? Would you eat them if they were prepared in a tasty and interesting way?

Plant chemicals are powerful agents for health. These substances act in our bodies to help reduce the incidence of cancer and other diseases. But how, we need to ask, do these phytochemicals affect the breast cells? By answering this vital question, we will be closer to an understanding of *why* the Five-a-Day for Better Health program can help alter your breast cancer risk profile in a positive manner; we will also know more about which fruits and vegetables hold the most promise of reducing the alarming rise in breast cancer rates in this country and elsewhere around the world.

In order to understand what medical research has revealed about this process, however, we need first to know more about the hormone estrogen and how it functions in a woman's body. This subject is explored in the next chapter.

PLANT FOODS IMPORTANT TO HUMAN NUTRITION

Family of Plants	Common Name	Comments
Cruciferous Vegetables (cabbage family)	Cabbage, Broccoli Brussels sprouts Cauliflower Collard, Kale Broccoli rabe Watercress Bitter cress Horseradish Turnip Radishes Swede, Rutabaga Bok choy Mustard seed	The whole cabbage family is well known for its anticancer properties, particularly against breast and colon cancer. Several varieties of cabbage exist, including savoy, green, and red. Many of the cruciferous vegetables, especially kale and the other greens, are rich in vitamin C, calcium, and vitamin A.
Umbelliferous Vegetables (carrot and parsley family)	Celery, Parsley, Fennel, Carrot, Parsnip, Dill, Coriander, Cumin, Caraway	Many of these umbelliferous plants are great sources of beta-carotene and vitamins A and C. The last four listed are generally used as herbs.

PLANT FOODS IMPORTANT TO HUMAN NUTRITION

Family of Plants	Common Name	Comments
Grains and Grasses	Wheat, Rye, Oats, Barley, Rice, Corn, Sorghum, Bulgur Buckwheat Wild rice Bamboo shoots Amaranth, Flax	These grains and grasses are excellent sources of soluble and insoluble fiber. Many contain abundant amounts of complex carbohydrates and B complex vitamins. Buckwheat is used traditionally in Italian polenta. Wild rice is a form of grass seed, not actually a rice. Amaranth and flax have recently become more popular as a source of carbohydrate and fiber.
Legumes (bean family)	Kidney beans Lima beans, Peas Soybeans Lupine beans Chickpeas Lentils String beans Carob, Peanut Mung beans	Literally thousands of varieties of legumes are known to exist. All are abundant sources of dietary fiber and protein. They are also a great source of the B vitamins. String beans are actually unripe versions of a hard bean. Carob is often used as a substitute for chocolate.
Leafy Green Vegetables	Chicory greens Belgian endive Radicchio Endive, Escarole Lettuce Dandelion greens Spinach Swiss chard Beet greens Arugula	Some of these leafy green vegetables may contain 3,000–8,000 IUs (international units) of vitamin A per serving. In addition, they contain abundant quantities of the B vitamins. All of these greens are easy to adapt to different recipes. For example, Swiss chard is a tasty alternative to spinach in some dishes.
Allium Vegetables (garlic/onion family)	Onion, Garlic, Shallots, Chives, Leek	The allium family of vegetables is also well known for its disease-preventing properties.
Potato Family	Potato, Tomato, Peppers, Eggplant	Some members of the potato family, such as tomatoes and peppers, are rich in carotenoid compounds. They are also a great source of vitamin C and other phytochemicals.

PLANT FOODS IMPORTANT TO HUMAN NUTRITION

Family of Plants	Common Name	Comments
Cucumber/Squash Family	Summer squash Winter squash Chayote Pumpkin Cucumber Watermelon Summer melons	Summer varieties of squash include zucchini, crookneck, and scallop. Popular winter varieties are acorn, butternut, spaghetti, and Hubbard. Many of these vegetables are incredibly rich in beta-carotene and vitamin A.
Miscellaneous Vegetables	Artichokes, Asparagus, Beets, Mushrooms, Taro root, Sweet potato, Yams, Olives, Capers, Water chestnut, Rhubarb, Ginger, Tea, Okra	Each of these miscellaneous vegetables has its own unique flavor and taste. Each contributes its own different phytochemicals to our diet. Note that sweet potatoes are much more abundant in vitamin A than yams. Actually, most yams sold in supermarkets are sweet potatoes; just remember, the more orange the better.
Fruits	Apple, Pear, Loquat, Medlar Plum, Cherry Peach, Nectarine Apricot, Quince Raspberry, Blackberry Gooseberry, Mulberry Currants, Grapes Huckleberry Figs, Dates Pomegranate Pineapple Avocado, Papaya Litchi, Mango Passion fruit Persimmon Kiwi fruit Prickly pear, Banana Citrus fruits Nuts Edible seeds	Nearly all fruits are rich sources of vitamin C, fiber, and potassium. Certain items, such as the kiwi fruit, have become more popular recently. Citrus fruits encompass a huge variety, including orange, citron, lemon, grapefruit, clementine, kumquat, and tangerine. Edible seeds include poppy seed, sesame seed, sunflower seed, and alfalfa seed.

CHAPTER SIX

THE ESTROGEN CONNECTION

Uncovering Estrogen's Link to Breast Cancer

In 1896, Dr. George T. Beatson, a surgeon in Glasgow, Scotland, performed an operation that marked the beginning of the history of breast cancer prevention. His results were published in a highly detailed report in the British medical journal *Lancet*. In his report, Beatson described the surgical treatment of two breast cancer patients, one a woman of forty, the other a woman of forty-nine. Both women suffered from advanced, incurable malignancies of the breast.

Dr. Beatson faced a difficult dilemma: How could he help these women? For both of them, the tumors were life-threatening. Based on their prior experience and observations, Beatson and his colleagues had begun to suspect that a woman's ovaries in some way fueled the growth of breast tumors. Acting on this clinical hunch, and in hope of possibly reducing stimulation to the breasts, Beatson operated on both patients to remove their ovaries and fallopian tubes. The surgery appeared to be successful. Both women left the

hospital in much less pain, leading Beatson to remark, "I am in-
clined to think that the disease is in a more quiescent stage and
gives some indication of a possible cure.

"The conclusion I draw from the two cases I have brought under
notice is this," he wrote, "that we must look in the female to the
ovaries as the seat of the exciting cause of carcinoma, certainly of
the mamma [breast], in all probability of the female generative
organs generally, and possibly of the rest of the body."

By removing the ovaries, Beatson had provided *the world's first
antiestrogen therapy* for breast cancer. The overall results, as outlined
in the hospital charts, were truly dramatic. Only nine days after
surgery, one of the patient's medical record states: "It was evident
that the cutaneous [skin] surface of the tumour was less vascular,
the red blush which covered it entirely being very noticeably dimin-
ished; while on October 14th [two days later] it was remarked that
the patient stated very emphatically of her own accord that she felt
'in a different world,' the pain in her breast being so much easier
as to be almost gone."

Beatson instantly recognized the value of this operation. "I know
that I have had nothing in the way of great results," he modestly
admitted, "but it must be remarked that I have worked with most
unpromising cases and that when large masses of cancer are present
it is not easy to bring healing influences to bear upon them. They
have got beyond control whereas in the early stage they might have
been amenable to treatment."

So gratifying were these results that by 1910 removal of the
ovaries was viewed as a helpful choice for many women with advanced breast tumors. Still, the basic question remained: What
was it about removing the ovaries that caused such a remarkable
remission for these women with malignant breast tumors?

An earlier clue to the crucial link between ovarian function and
breast cancer had actually emerged nearly two centuries earlier. An
Italian physician, Bernardino Ramazzini, had published studies in
1700, in which he noted an unusually high incidence of breast
tumors among Roman Catholic nuns. He suggested their cloistered

celibate lives contributed to the disease and remarked, "You seldom find a convent that does not harbor this accursed pest, cancer, within its walls."

This association was later confirmed by a separate study of nuns whose deaths were recorded in the city of Verona between 1760 and 1839. The menstrual cycles of a celibate woman normally continue without interruption until menopause. Her ovaries undergo an *estrogen surge* month after month, from her teenage years until menopause.

Dr. Beatson's observations made it clear that the ovaries were indeed linked to breast cancer. Nevertheless, it took the next two decades for chemists to establish the existence of steroid hormones in the body, including estrogen.

During a woman's menstrual cycle, the ovaries compete with each other to generate a single egg to undergo ovulation. As the day of ovulation draws near, the ovaries begin to produce large amounts of estrogen in order to prepare the uterus for a possible pregnancy. This monthly surge of estrogen occurs over and over again throughout a woman's reproductive life and is therefore the crucial link to breast cancer.

It was noted by surgeons, however, that removal of the ovaries in older women did not have the same beneficial effects against breast tumors. As endocrinologists learned to measure the minute levels of hormones in the body, they discovered that estrogen is still present in older women, though at very low levels. In postmenopausal women, the adrenal glands become the source of large quantities of estrogen building blocks, converted in fat cells to active estrogen. Thus, removal of the adrenal glands provided another hopeful alternative for alleviating the suffering of older women with breast cancer.

Once again, the common denominator of these therapies was the *removal of estrogen*. Ever since Dr. Beatson's time, it has become increasingly clear that estrogen plays a crucial role in both the development and the continued growth of malignant breast cells. But what exactly is estrogen? How does it act in the breasts?

The Estrogen Pathway

Estrogens are members of a family of chemicals in the body called *steroid hormones*. The term *estrogen* actually refers to several closely related compounds, all derived from the principal estrogen in a woman's body, *estradiol*. These different forms of estrogen are believed by researchers to be critically important in the causation of breast tumors.

Estrogens are but one of the classes of steroid hormones important to a woman's health. Other groups of steroid hormones include:

- progesterone—a female steroid important for pregnancy
- testosterone—a sex steroid present in men, and in lesser amounts in women
- cortisol—a steroid involved in immune functions
- vitamin D—a modified steroid important to bones
- aldosterone—a steroid that acts in the kidneys to control sodium balance

Over the years, scientists have discovered that all of these steroid hormones share two important traits: They are produced in extremely small amounts and they act only in *specific tissues* of the body. Each of them is important to a woman's good health.

Too much of a good thing, however, can sometimes be as harmful as too little. This is the paradox of estrogen. Medical scientists have learned a great deal more in recent decades about the dangerous effects of *excessive amounts of estrogen* and the sinister role estrogen plays in stimulating the growth of breast cells.

Our own research, published in the *Journal of the National Cancer Institute*, has shown that certain forms of estrogen can actually attack healthy breast cells, increasing the cell's risk of devastating DNA changes. Estrogen alone, therefore, may sometimes act as the *primary* catalyst for a malignant breast tumor.

The production, activity, breakdown, and elimination of estrogen in a woman's body may be conceptualized as four steps of a single biological process or pathway. We call this the Estrogen

Pathway. The steps of the Estrogen Pathway can be outlined as follows:

THE ESTROGEN PATHWAY:

1. Estrogen is produced in the body.
2. Estrogen circulates throughout the body.
3. Estrogen binds to the estrogen receptor.
4. Estrogen is broken down and eliminated.

Let us see what actually happens to estrogen in a woman's body at each of these four steps.

First: *Estrogen is produced in the body.* In women, most estrogen production takes place in the ovaries. Estrogen production begins at about twelve to fourteen years of age and continues until menopause at about fifty to fifty-five years of age. Even after menopause, however, estrogen still continues to be produced. In older women, fat and muscle tissue become the main organs for manufacturing estrogen, using the hormonal building blocks supplied by the adrenal glands, as described earlier.

Second: *Estrogen circulates throughout the body,* generally moving in the bloodstream from the ovaries or the fat cells to the breasts (and other organs). This circulation system uses a carrier molecule in the blood called *sex hormone–binding globulin,* or *SHBG.* This carrier molecule attaches to estrogen in the bloodstream once it is produced, then transports the estrogen hormone to other cells able to use it.

Third: *Estrogen binds to the estrogen receptor* in breast cells. This is an extremely important process by which estrogen is "captured" from the bloodstream by a specialized cell protein able to *recognize only estrogen.* The estrogen receptors are present within cells of several tissues of a woman's body. Most are found in the breasts and the uterus, with lesser amounts in the skin, bone, brain, and liver.

Once an active estrogen molecule binds to the estrogen receptor, that cell's DNA becomes activated. As a result, the cell may grow. This process can be compared to a car engine's lock and key: An estrogen hormone acts like the key, the estrogen receptor is the lock, and the cell's DNA is like the engine. Once the key (estrogen) is inserted, the lock (receptor) is opened and the engine turns on (DNA is activated).

Fourth: *Estrogen is broken down and eliminated*, a process scientists call metabolism. Once estrogen has done its work, it is chemically changed (or metabolized) in order to help the body eliminate it. Estrogen by-products, or metabolites, are excreted from the body through the urine and intestines. While urinary estrogen is completely eliminated, some of the intestinal estrogens are recycled and returned to the bloodstream for further hormonal activity.

Work begun at The Rockefeller University Hospital in New York City and continued at the Foundation's Institute for Hormone Research demonstrated that two major by-products are formed during the breakdown of estrogen. These are referred to as *the C-16 metabolite* and *the C-2 metabolite*. (Figure 6 shows that C-2 and C-16 differ only in the location of a single -OH metabolic change.)

We found a crucial difference between these two estrogen metabolites: C-16 seems to remain active as a hormone in a woman's body, while the C-2 form is essentially inactive.

Our published studies revealed that C-16 is able to attack DNA and cause abnormal growth of breast cells. Women with breast cancer formed excessive amounts of the C-16 estrogen, as reported in the *Proceedings of the National Academy of Sciences*. In addition, we found that women from families with a history of breast cancer also had elevated formation of C-16 estrogen.

Our latest studies have *uncovered substances in common fruits and vegetables* capable of reducing the formation of the potentially dangerous C-16 estrogen metabolite in a woman's body. These plant substances encourage the production of safer, inactive C-2 forms of the hormone.

Our research has made it clear that *each* of the four steps of the Estrogen Pathway can be modified by phytochemicals in foods you *could be eating* today. You will soon learn how several elements of a *traditional diet and lifestyle* combine to reduce the risks estrogen poses for the abnormal growth of breast cells.

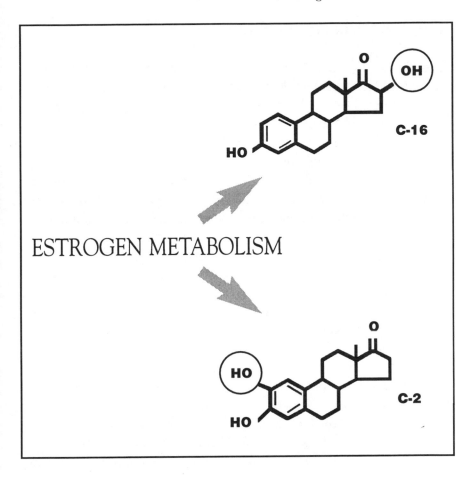

ESTROGEN METABOLISM

FIGURE 6

Striving Toward a Healthy Estrogen Balance

In general, a woman's body tries to maintain a balance of estrogen activity that is neither too low nor too high. A system of hormonal checks and balances usually operates smoothly and silently. This delicate balance becomes evident only when the levels are insufficient or excessive.

Conditions Linked to Insufficient Estrogen

Estrogen hormones play a vital role in many different aspects of a woman's life, most notably in human sexuality and reproduction. Estrogen manufactured by the ovaries is critical for the precise timing of the release of the egg each month. If hormonal levels fall too low, an egg may not be released, leading to infertility and its often tragic emotional consequences.

Inadequate levels of estrogen can also become evident in other ways. Estrogen is necessary, for example, in the growth of the lining of the uterus (the endometrium). Each month, the endometrial lining is made ready to receive a fertilized egg and to help build a nourishing placenta for a potential pregnancy. If estrogen levels fall too low in a woman's body, the uterus will not be properly stimulated to grow and develop. Menstruation eventually ceases and pregnancy is no longer possible. In addition, when estrogen levels are too low, the vagina can no longer provide its own lubrication, resulting in painful sexual intercourse.

Another reproductive function of estrogen is to promote the growth and development of breast tissue, helping to ensure that milk production will be adequate to nurse an infant. Estrogen is also necessary for the health of the skin. These hormones encourage the formation of collagen, a natural protein that provides the structural support for all skin cells. When collagen production decreases, the skin becomes thin and less supple.

Two other important parts of a woman's body that are dependent upon adequate supplies of estrogen are the bones and the blood vessels. Bone cells have been found to contain estrogen receptors. These receptors respond favorably to the abundant hormone levels present during the reproductive years of a woman's life by encouraging the formation of dense, calcium-rich bones.

By age thirty-five, a woman's bones are about as thick and strong as they will ever be. If, however, estrogen is severely reduced early in life, premature loss of precious bone calcium may occur. Osteoporosis, a condition of weak and brittle bones, may be the eventual result. Osteoporosis resulting from chronically low estrogen levels leaves women vulnerable to fractures of the hips, arms, and spine.

Estrogen is also largely responsible for the protection against heart disease women enjoy for much of their lives. It helps the heart by encouraging the formation of HDL cholesterol, called "good" cholesterol, known to keep blood vessels free of atherosclerosis (hardening of the arteries).

CONDITIONS LINKED TO AN ESTROGEN IMBALANCE

LACK OF ESTROGEN	EXCESSIVE ESTROGEN
Osteoporosis	Proliferative breast disease
Cessation of menses	(dense breasts)
Infertility	Irregular or excessive menses
Premature menopause	Breast and uterine cancer
Hot flashes, vaginal dryness	Endometriosis

Conditions Linked to Excessive Estrogen

While some women may have too little estrogen, others may have too much. Some tissues, such as the bones, benefit from an abundance of estrogen; others, such as the breasts and uterus, may not. Estrogen causes breast cells to multiply. Over time, this ongoing growth of breast tissue can lead to dense breasts, a condition visible on a woman's mammogram.

Mammographic breast densities were recently compared between young Japanese women and a comparable group of British women by an international team of scientists. Their report showed the breasts of Japanese women were much less dense, indicating less breast cell growth. This finding remained significant, even when the researchers ruled out such things as later onset of menstruation, earlier childbirth, and lower body weights of the Japanese women.

Interestingly, an earlier study in 1979 had found little difference in the mammogram densities among a large group of women living in Hawaii, regardless of whether they were of Caucasian, Japanese, or Chinese ancestry. Presumably, the protective effect on breast cell growth previously enjoyed in Japan or China was lost soon after these women moved to Hawaii and adopted a more Western diet and lifestyle.

Is the increased density of the breasts in Western women related to higher estrogen levels? The answer is yes. Scientific evidence suggests that estrogen is a critical piece of the breast cancer puzzle. Estrogen can set up a breast cell for the greater likelihood of a dangerous gene mutation by *boosting cell division*, thereby heightening the chance for a mutation in that cell's DNA.

The extra growth of breast cells caused by excessive estrogen may be particularly dangerous under certain conditions. For example, the DNA's normal wear and tear may not be fully repaired if the cells are dividing too rapidly. In rapidly growing cells, a chance mutation may occur in one of the dangerous tumor-suppressor genes, which undoubtedly could spell disaster for the breasts.

Estrogen Plays a Role in Many of the Risk Factors

If we consider all of the known or suspected risks for breast cancer, *we find that abnormal or excessive estrogen activity is implicated in many of them.* Let us review the risk factors presented in Chapter 2 to see which ones involve estrogen.

The dangerous role played by estrogen in many of these risk factors is clear. Both early menarche and late menopause, for example, can potentially be linked to a greater number of menstrual cycles throughout a woman's life. Each menstrual cycle involves another monthly surge, bathing the breast cells in estrogen.

Some women in families prone to breast cancer inherit a ten-

INVOLVEMENT OF ESTROGEN IN THE KNOWN RISK FACTORS FOR BREAST CANCER

Risk Category	Increased Risk	Estrogen Involved?
Reproductive Factors		
Early menarche	1.3	Yes
Late first birth or no children	1.9	
Late menopause	1.5	Yes
No breast-feeding	1.2	
Individual and Genetic Factors		
Positive family history of breast cancer	2.5	Yes
Benign breast disease	2.5	Yes
Height	1.3	
Age (see page 35)		
Environmental Factors		
Oral contraceptives	1.5	Yes
Estrogen replacement therapy	2.1	Yes
Alcohol	2.0	Yes
Radiation	1.5	
Pesticide exposure	2.0	Yes
Lifestyle Factors		
Diet	1.5 or greater	Yes
Lack of exercise	1.3	Yes
Obesity	1.5	Yes

dency to produce abnormally high levels of the dangerous C-16 form of estrogen. Women with malignant breast tumors have been found to form the C-16 estrogen at *double the rate* of healthy women. The daughters of women with breast tumors were also found to produce higher amounts of these dangerous estrogens.

Benign breast disease is dangerous because of the increased growth and proliferation of breast cells associated with this condition. The greatest stimulus for the excessive growth of breast cells is estrogen. Additional amounts of this hormone taken into the body, either in the form of oral contraceptives early in life or as postmenopausal estrogen replacement therapy later in life can further stimulate the growth of breast cells.

The effects of alcohol and pesticides on estrogen metabolism are complex and poorly understood. Alcohol is known to be toxic to some cells in the body and possibly to the cells of the breasts. It has at least two effects on the body's estrogen hormones. One recent study showed that estrogen concentrations in the urine rose quickly when women had at least two drinks of alcohol each day on a regular basis. It has also been found to suppress the formation of the favorable C-2 estrogen, thereby further robbing the breasts of protection.

Pesticides are also believed to affect the metabolism of estrogen in the body adversely. Some pesticides have been found to activate the estrogen receptor, thereby stimulating the breasts just like supplemental estrogen. This may explain the increased malignancies of the breasts in women exposed to high levels of these toxic substances. In addition to effects on estrogen, many pesticides may also be toxic to the cell's DNA.

Diet has a profound effect on the Estrogen Pathway in a woman's body. It can influence each of the four steps of this pathway. The effects of the foods you eat on this hormonal process are discussed in detail below.

Exercise stimulates the inactivation of estrogen by *raising C-2 estrogen formation*. This fact was shown in the studies of Dr. Rose Frisch and her colleagues at Harvard University, cited earlier. Dr. Frisch's team showed how the lower risk associated with exercise is related to leanness and the effects of low body fat on estrogen metabolism.

Excessive body fat also exerts three dangerous effects on the body's estrogen. First, *fat cells are factories for producing estrogen* (recall the first step of the Estrogen Pathway). This effect is particularly serious for postmenopausal obese women. Second, obesity strongly suppresses the formation of the favorable C-2 estrogen metabolite (step four).

Third, some forms of obesity (especially when more body fat is located above the waist) lower the circulating level of the important sex hormone–binding protein, or SHBG (step two of the pathway). Without enough SHBG present to keep the estrogen in the bloodstream, greater amounts of the hormone are able to travel directly *into breast cells* and stimulate growth. This dangerous scenario may help to explain the greater rates of breast and uterine malignancies observed in some women with upper-body obesity.

Can the Dangers of Estrogen Be Reduced?

The general acceptance by the scientific community of the role of estrogen in fueling breast tumors has come about slowly. Recent research evidence, however, has made this case much stronger.

Nearly twenty years ago, prominent researchers led by Dr. Brian MacMahon of the Harvard University School of Public Health began to consider the evidence for this relationship. As early as 1973, Dr. MacMahon stated, "*The most credible working hypothesis at present is that relating breast cancer risk to estrogen metabolism.*" His conclusion was based on the strong evidence linking breast cancer and the ovaries.

Since that time, estrogen has been scrutinized by researchers all over the world as a potential cause of breast malignancies. While some scientists are still not convinced estrogen can actually *cause* breast cancer, no one disputes the fact that estrogen *encourages* the growth of malignant breast cells once they arise.

As we learned in Chapter 3, enormous changes in diet and

lifestyle took place in Japanese women after World War II. These changes reduced the hormonal differences between Japanese women and those women living in such high-risk countries as England and the United States. Cancer researchers, therefore, turned their attention to China, where millions of women continue to follow a largely traditional diet and lifestyle.

An initial research study measured estrogen in blood samples collected from 3,250 rural Chinese women living in sixty-five different counties and compared them with similar measurements in a group of 300 British women. The researchers found estrogen levels were *much lower* in the Chinese women at all ages studied. This is particularly important in light of the fact that breast cancer rates in China are one-fifth or less than rates in Western countries.

This same research team also studied blood-estrogen levels in an urban population of young Chinese women living in Shanghai and compared them with urban women in Los Angeles. The Chinese women *still had lower estrogen levels*, suggesting that urban Chinese continue to maintain a diet that is largely protective. Obviously fast food and rich ice cream have not yet made deep inroads into mainland China, even in the cities. There's only one McDonald's so far in Beijing, even though it is the world's largest.

The latest evidence of the estrogen link to breast cancer was uncovered by Dr. Paolo Toniolo at New York University. For the past eight years, Dr. Toniolo has directed the NYU Women's Health Study, in which over sixteen thousand women were enrolled in advance and were then tracked for the occurrence of breast tumors over time. Multiple blood samples were collected from all the women and carefully frozen.

Dr. Toniolo has reported that in the group of older postmenopausal women he studied, higher estrogen levels were strongly associated with a greater risk of developing a breast malignancy in later years. His findings are thus far among the strongest data linking excessive estrogen to future breast malignancies.

Many breast cancer researchers have reached an important conclusion: *If breast cancer rates are to be reduced, it will be necessary to lower the excessive stimulatory effects of estrogen throughout the popula-*

tion, *particularly in those women at higher risk.* This conclusion represents an enormous challenge to the medical and research communities. Is it possible to limit safely the actions of estrogen without causing a woman harm?

The answer, many physicians believe, is *yes.* And since there are four steps to the Estrogen Pathway, there may even be several ways to do so. Many different chemicals, natural and synthetic, may reduce the dangerous actions of estrogen in a woman's breasts. The most exciting news is that some of these anticancer chemicals are found in the plant foods we eat.

MINIMIZING THE DANGEROUS EFFECTS OF ESTROGEN

Medical researchers have long concluded that estrogen plays a critical role in promoting the growth of breast tumors. It is also becoming clear that estrogen itself may damage a breast cell's DNA, thus *causing* breast cancer in some women. Therefore, scientists have begun to turn their attention to ways of safely reducing the action of this hormone in women's bodies in the hope of reducing breast cancer rates.

We know, however, that estrogen cannot be eliminated *entirely* in a healthy young woman without dangerous consequences. Can we, then, limit the actions of this hormone in a safe way? The answer is an emphatic *yes*. An understanding of the Estrogen Pathway suggests ways to reduce the adverse effects of estrogen in the female body. The Estrogen Pathway, as you will recall, consists of four steps (see page 81).

Researchers are currently investigating several chemicals that can act directly upon the Estrogen Pathway to reduce the stimulating effect of this hormone. These research efforts are the historical continuation of the pioneering work of Beatson and others to reduce the dangerous effects of estrogen on breast cells.

Two experimental trials currently in progress involve the drugs tamoxifen and LHRHa. It is hoped that these drugs will benefit women at high risk for breast cancer. Tamoxifen is a synthetic hormone used as a chemotherapeutic agent in the treatment of breast cancer. Another synthetic hormone primarily used in the treatment of endometriosis is LHRHa, which stands for *luteinizing hormone releasing hormone agonist*. This compound is modeled after LHRH, a pituitary hormone.

Pharmaceutical Approaches to Blocking the Action of Estrogen

Prevention of Breast Cancer Using Tamoxifen

Tamoxifen was originally developed in 1966 as part of a search for agents useful in the treatment of cancer. This hormonelike drug was soon found to be effective in treating women with breast cancers. Rather than killing cells, however, scientists discovered tamoxifen worked by *blocking* estrogen's ability to bind to the estrogen receptor. It acts, therefore, by interrupting step three of the Estrogen Pathway. Since tamoxifen interferes with the receptor, a woman's breast cells are unable to detect the natural estrogens in her body. Breast cells, therefore, *starve* from lack of estrogen, leading to the shrinkage of many breast tumors.

This hormone blocker does not kill cells, as other chemotherapeutic agents do. It, therefore, has little of the toxicity normally associated with drugs used in treating cancer. Over the past twenty-five years, countless women have been given the drug as part of their chemotherapy. Many clinicians and research scientists have come to see tamoxifen as one of the most important breakthroughs for women with breast cancer. In early 1992, a detailed analysis of all of the different treatment choices facing women with breast cancer was reported in the British journal *Lancet*; it concluded that tamoxifen was unrivaled in the treatment of breast tumors, especially among women over the age of sixty.

As a result of tamoxifen's success in treating women with breast cancer, an even more intriguing potential use of the drug soon came to light. Women with a history of breast cancer face a greater chance of developing a *second* tumor in the other breast. Tamoxifen seemed to be able to prevent this second breast tumor in some women.

Scientists compared nearly five thousand women who had received the drug following their first encounter with breast cancer with a comparable number of breast cancer patients who *never* used it as part of their treatment. The results were exciting: The researchers were able to show a 35 percent decrease in second cancers of the other breast among women who had used tamoxifen.

This finding led some physicians to ask whether tamoxifen might also prevent breast tumors in healthy women who had not yet developed the disease. If this drug was indeed as safe as it appeared to be, they reasoned, then perhaps it could eventually be taken as a preventive agent by high-risk women early in life.

Breast cancer researchers therefore faced two important tasks: first, to determine *whether tamoxifen will be truly effective* as a preventive measure; second, *to establish its safety* for long-term use by healthy women.

The National Cancer Institute has funded a large national research trial to address the question of tamoxifen's effectiveness as a preventive agent. The tamoxifen trial, begun in 1992, will be conducted as a double-blinded trial over the next eight years, during which time eight thousand women will receive the actual drug, while another eight thousand will receive a placebo.

Despite the criticism this project has drawn, its approval clearly demonstrates broad scientific support for breast cancer prevention strategies that are *based upon minimizing the stimulatory action of estrogen in healthy women.* The answer to the question of tamoxifen's effectiveness in preventing breast tumors will not be known until the trial's completion eight years hence.

The second question—Is it safe?—has generated considerable controversy in itself. Tamoxifen has been used since the early 1970s by hundreds of thousands of women with breast cancer. Most oncologists and patients believe that it has shown relatively little toxicity in these women.

The perspective of a woman with breast cancer, however, is quite different from that of a healthy woman, particularly as to what constitutes a *serious* side effect. Tamoxifen is known to cause nausea in about 5 to 10 percent of women using it, and depression in around 1 percent of patients. Symptoms such as hot flashes, facial flushing, irregular periods, decreased sexual desire, and vaginal discharge have all been reported by some women on the drug. In fact, one or more of these side effects are usually experienced by one out of five women taking tamoxifen. Up to 10 percent of women in scientific studies of tamoxifen have been forced to drop out because of these problems.

But these side effects are still not considered serious by the many women who have used tamoxifen regularly to treat their breast tumors. For these women, the drug is an acceptable alternative to more conventional and more toxic chemotherapeutic agents. Thus, the question remains: Would these same kinds of side effects be acceptable to a *healthy young woman* trying to lessen her risk of this terrible disease?

There are three other potential side effects of concern to healthy women using tamoxifen. First, there is the possibility of deep vein thrombosis, which refers to a blood clot of the large veins of the leg and pelvis. In the small number of patients who develop such a thrombosis, there is a risk that the blood clot will travel to the lungs, which is potentially fatal.

Second, it is likely some of the women using tamoxifen will develop uterine cancer as a result of the drug, even at the lower doses used in the U.S. trial. The risk of a uterine malignancy from tamoxifen is similar to that associated with the use of estrogen replacement therapy by postmenopausal women. In a 1989 tamoxifen trial conducted in Stockholm, for example, 13 out of 931 women on this drug developed uterine cancer, compared with only 2 out of 915 women who didn't receive it.

Some physicians have argued that uterine cancer is not nearly as dangerous to women as breast cancer, and they maintain that it will occur infrequently on the lower dosages given in the U.S. tamoxifen trial. Women who are carefully checked by their gynecologists and undergo regular endometrial biopsies face little risk of dying from a uterine tumor. But critics of the tamoxifen trial take small comfort in such reassurances. To Dr. Adrian Fugh-Berman, a physician adviser to the National Women's Health Network, this argument sounds a lot like disease substitution, which she and other women's health advocates do not favor.

Finally, according to the Swedish research studies, there is a small risk of liver cancer from the use of tamoxifen. Scientists have begun to examine liver damage in animals receiving this drug. According to recent published studies, substantial amounts of DNA damage can be detected. But at this time, no one fully knows the risk for fatal liver cancers from long-term use of tamoxifen by healthy women.

Despite these concerns, the tamoxifen trial is meeting its patient recruitment goals. As of December 1992, the *Journal of the National Cancer Institute* reported that over twenty thousand women had applied and many provisionally accepted into the study.

Prevention of Breast Cancer Using LHRHa

The second research trial under way among a small group of fourteen healthy women focuses on the drug LHRHa. LHRHa acts in a woman's body just like a powerful pituitary hormone, which normally controls the production of estrogen. It acts, therefore, by interrupting step one of the Estrogen Pathway.

LHRHa causes the ovaries to stop ovulating, thereby halting the production of ovarian hormones. The ovaries will return to normal shortly after the drug is discontinued. Scientists believe LHRHa will protect young women just as if they had had their ovaries temporarily removed. The research team performing the study believes breast cancer rates could be reduced as much as 70 percent in users of LHRHa. As with tamoxifen, many years will be needed before researchers know whether this approach is truly safe and effective.

Since estrogen levels fall very low as a result of LHRHa, women participating in this research trial have begun to experience bone loss and other symptoms of estrogen deficiency. Therefore, the study design also involves a complicated arrangement of hormones *given back* to the patient. These include a low-dose estrogen-containing oral contraceptive pill taken for twenty-one- out of every twenty-eight-day period and a progesterone supplement taken for twelve days every three to four months. The progesterone is needed to cause menstruation, thereby replacing the uterine lining on a regular basis.

The LHRHa trial is still small and highly experimental, and it will involve at most only a few women. This trial, however, also underscores *the growing scientific acceptance of reducing the action of estrogen* as a means to prevent breast cancer.

Finding Anti-Breast Cancer Agents in the Foods You Eat

Results from the research trials just discussed will probably not be available to the public until the next century. Furthermore, drug approaches may be too complicated or hazardous for most women. In either case, these strategies are simply not applicable to women at average risk for developing breast cancer.

Whether tamoxifen can ever be used by healthy young women over a period of many years for the prevention of breast cancer is uncertain. This important drug has increased the quality of life for thousands of women diagnosed with breast cancer. For these women, tamoxifen represents a major defense against the return of their tumors. They and we are grateful for the hope it offers.

Nevertheless, even if tamoxifen eventually is proven to be a safe and effective agent in the prevention of breast cancer, all women would still benefit by making *dietary changes* that can further lower their risk. While tamoxifen blocks the third step of the Estrogen Pathway—the binding of estrogen to its receptor—dietary change holds out the promise of affecting all four steps of the pathway safely.

Many of the foods we could include in our diets are a source of breast-healthy phytochemicals. Some of these plant compounds possess properties remarkably similar to the drugs Tamoxifen and LHRHa. We believe it was these plant substances, and not only the lower levels of fat, that contributed to the positive outcome of the Women's Health Trial.

Because plant chemicals are already being eaten daily, to some extent, by hundreds of millions of women around the world, we know that they are generally safe. In the next chapter, we will discuss this natural pharmacy and *why* it can help to reduce breast cancers in healthy women.

BREAST CANCER-FIGHTING PHYTOCHEMICALS

The Five-a-Day for Better Health program proposed by the NCI is based on the scientific conclusion that a diet that includes at least five servings of a variety of vegetables and fruits each day will help reduce your risk of developing cancer. As we have just seen from the two surveys of scientific research into the relationship of diet and cancer, study after study found cancer rates reduced in those women and men eating the largest amounts of fruits and vegetables. Medical researchers have concluded that the phytochemicals in these foods can also provide a helpful, relatively simple way to reduce the risk of breast cancer.

Knowledge of this powerful cancer-protection process comes from in-depth research of many different phytochemicals found in particular fruits and vegetables. These clinical studies have been carried out by research teams around the world, each examining specific substances in certain plants.

Research studies at our Institute for Hormone Research have centered upon the cruciferous family of vegetables, specifically on a class of phytochemicals they contain called *indoles*. Our laboratory has performed intensive testing of one of these compounds, indole-3-carbinol, or *I-3-C*. While many of our findings are still preliminary, we believe that indoles and some other plant chemicals could actually reduce the growth of abnormal breast cells in women.

Indoles and Related Compounds in the Cabbage Family

The unique chemical makeup of the cruciferous family of vegetables was studied as early as the 1940s by researchers in Finland. Yet it was not until thirty years later that Dr. Lee Wattenberg, a professor at the University of Minnesota, focused attention on their unique cancer-fighting properties.

In animal experiments, Dr. Wattenberg learned that animals eating diets supplemented with broccoli, brussels sprouts, or cabbage developed far fewer breast tumors than animals that were not fed the cruciferous vegetables. His pioneering research was quickly noticed by dozens of other scientists around the world, who confirmed his exciting discoveries.

Dr. Wattenberg paid particular attention to three groups of phytochemicals in the cabbage family, including indoles. He was able to show that feeding experimental animals one compound in particular, I-3-C, had roughly the same cancer-fighting effects as if they ate the whole vegetable.

It was Dr. Wattenberg's remarkable observation that eventually opened the door for our own laboratory studies of cabbage compounds and breast cancer prevention in women. My colleagues and I posed a critical question: Would eating these cruciferous compounds have a beneficial effect on the estrogen in a woman's body? To answer this, we decided to study the effect of phytochemical *I-3-C* on estrogen metabolism in women.

We focused our efforts on changes in the fourth step of the estrogen pathway—the breakdown and elimination of estrogen. As mentioned earlier, we already knew that there are basically two types of estrogen formed during the breakdown process: the *active* C-16 form and the *inactive* C-2 form. C-16 estrogens were found to cause mutations in breast cells, and they were formed at much faster rates in women with breast cancer, as well as in those women at higher risk for the disease. For example, women from families with breast cancer, obese women, women doing little aerobic exercise, and women eating high-fat diets all showed greater formation of C-16 estrogen in their bodies. On the other hand, the inactive C-2 estrogens were produced in larger amounts in women whose breast cancer risk was lower.

Therefore, we developed the following hypothesis. *The consumption of cruciferous vegetables, or purified I-3-C, may reduce breast cell growth and breast cancer by encouraging the transformation of a woman's estrogens into the inactive, safer C-2 form.*

Our initial test of this hypothesis showed that this indeed was the case. A series of experiments were designed to critically evaluate the use of I-3-C as a breast cancer preventive agent. Our first study examined the use of I-3-C in animals. The results of our study were published in the journal *Carcinogenesis.* We reported that the cabbage compound led directly to a reduction in the number and size of breast tumors in mice.

Building upon the results of our animal experiments, we investigated the use of I-3-C itself in healthy women, many of whom were at high risk for breast cancer. These women took I-3-C for varying periods of time, lasting from one week to three months. None of the seventy-five women who participated in these studies experienced any significant side effects from I-3-C.

As we reported in the *Journal of the National Cancer Institute,* women volunteers who took pure I-3-C daily doubled their production of C-2 estrogens. Moreover, they reduced the amount of C-16 estrogens in their bodies, as well. In another as-yet-unpublished study, we found that the biochemical effects of I-3-C remained steady for the entire three-month period of testing. These results tell us that the beneficial effects of I-3-C continue over an extended period of time.

Larger clinical studies of indole-3-carbinol are under way. It will take time, however, to understand fully how physicians can use this and other phytochemicals directly in women. Unfortunately, such phytochemical studies proceed only as fast as research funds permit. According to a recent *New York Times* article by science writer Natalie Angier, "*On average only about 5 percent of the approximately $1.8 billion annual budget of the National Cancer Institute has been earmarked for disease prevention,* [italics mine] with far more going toward expensive and high profile studies like those on gene therapy, which if it works, will take years before it is of any use to many cancer patients."

If purified I-3-C appears to be of such benefit, you may well ask yourself, Shouldn't I be taking it now? At this early stage in our research, the answer can only be a firm *no.* Precisely because I-3-C *does* alter hormonal metabolism so decisively, we are concerned that it may have other unknown properties. For example, it might adversely affect the metabolism of helpful substances in the body. Purified I-3-C should be viewed as a drug, not a food. The Food and Drug Administration has set a high standard for scientific research in the field of nutritional chemoprevention. Carefully designed clinical trials will need to be conducted to ensure the safe use of this compound.

It is our position, therefore, that women should not be encouraged to take any food or vitamin supplement containing purified indole-3-carbinol at this time. Women should not be misled by products whose promotional materials cite our published I-3-C research to lend authority to their claims.

There is another good reason to discourage the use of purified I-3-C supplements at this time. By relying solely on a supplement containing a single phytochemical, you would not be receiving the benefits of the other valuable plant compounds in crucifers. As mentioned earlier, Dr. Wattenberg originally pointed out that cruciferous vegetables contain three major classes of cancer-fighting phytochemicals. Another of these compounds in crucifers is sulforaphane. This particular phytochemical was recently described in a widely publicized series of experiments published by Dr. Paul Talalay of Johns Hopkins University School of Medicine.

Dr. Talalay and his colleagues discovered that sulforaphane, particularly abundant in broccoli, greatly stimulates the activity of several key enzymes whose job is to inactivate potentially toxic substances we might eat or breathe. When we eat cabbage or broccoli, we gain the benefits of *all* of these phytochemicals: I-3-C, sulforaphane, and others. A single purified agent simply does not provide all of these protective phytochemicals.

Based on the large body of cruciferous research, therefore, we can offer you the following suggestions for obtaining high amounts of these natural cancer-fighting phytochemicals in your diet. Let us review again the major members of the cruciferous family of vegetables.

Family of Plants	Common Name
Cruciferous	Cabbage
Vegetables	Broccoli
(cabbage	Brussels
family)	sprouts
	Cauliflower
	Collard,
	Kale
	Broccoli rabe
	Watercress
	Bitter cress
	Horseradish
	Turnip
	Radishes
	Swede,
	Rutabaga
	Bok choy
	Mustard seed

Indoles are heat-sensitive chemicals. Therefore, you should avoid overcooking any of the cabbage-family vegetables. Instead, steam them lightly or stir-fry them quickly using small amounts of vegetable oil. Whenever possible, eat these vegetables raw for the maximum health benefit.

Two crucifers with perhaps the greatest amounts of indoles are savoy cabbage (crinkly green leaves) and brussels sprouts. Rather than focusing on just one or two members of this family, however, it would be best to eat a wide variety of crucifers to obtain the greatest benefit.

It has been estimated that Japanese and Chinese women average well over one hundred milligrams of indoles each day by eating large amounts of several varieties of cabbage-family vegetables. By comparison, most American women average only twenty milligrams daily.

In order to approach the amounts eaten by Asian women, a good place to start is to *eat one or more servings of cruciferous vegetables at least three times each week.* During a typical week, for example, eat one or more servings of coleslaw (made using a low-fat salad dressing rather than high-fat mayonnaise). Serve lightly steamed cabbage, broccoli, brussels sprouts, or cauliflower each week. Serve sliced Chinese or red cabbage in a salad. Add sliced radishes or watercress to your tossed greens with a low-fat spicy dressing.

Most Americans do not take full advantage of the nutritional benefits of the cabbage-family greens. These include broccoli rabe, collard greens, kale, and turnip greens. Besides the indoles and some other unique phytochemicals present only in the cabbage family, these dark green vegetables also contain an abundance of vitamin A, beta-carotene, and other carotenoid compounds. While many greens are somewhat bitter, each of these vegetables can be enjoyed by simply sautéing lightly with a touch of olive oil and garlic.

Isoflavones in Soybeans

Soybeans are rich in several phytochemicals, many of which are believed to offer remarkable health benefits. These soy-derived phytochemicals include isoflavones, phytates, saponins, sterols, and protease inhibitors. All of these compounds may contribute to the soybean's anticancer arsenal. We will focus our attention on only one group, the isoflavones.

The importance of isoflavone phytochemicals in soybeans was discovered in the early 1970s. Researchers measuring the urinary levels of soybean isoflavones in Asian women found them to be thirty to one hundred times higher than in most American women. The higher levels of this phytochemical reflected the greater dietary intake of soybean-based products among Asian women.

Soy researchers soon made another critical finding: *The isoflavones in soybeans resemble the breast cancer-fighting drug tamoxifen.* Soy isoflavones share an ability to interact with the estrogen receptor (step three of the Estrogen Pathway). Because of this ability, isoflavones are also called plant estrogens or phytoestrogens.

How then do isoflavones potentially protect women against breast cancer? Since soy isoflavones are so much weaker than the natural estrogen hormones, they interfere with the receptor's functions without actually *triggering the receptor* in the breast. Using the lock-and-key analogy once again, isoflavone molecules (similar to estrogen) insert themselves into the lock (the receptor) but do not open it (activate DNA). As a result of this interference, the normal action of estrogen in a woman's breast appears to be lessened.

This discovery helps to explain the relationship between the consumption of soy-based foods in Asian countries and their lower rates of breast cancer. Laboratory experiments have confirmed this protective link. Researchers found, for example, that adding purified isoflavones from soybeans directly to human breast cancer cells in the laboratory reduced their rate of growth.

Soybean researchers have estimated that Asian women commonly eat well over thirty-five grams of soybeans, in one form or another, *each day*. This is equivalent to more than 150 milligrams of isoflavones. By comparison, most American women routinely eat less than one or two grams of soy products each day.

Most soybeans consumed by Americans are included in food

products for nonnutritional reasons. Soy protein concentrates, for example, are used by food manufacturers as texturizing, gelling, emulsifying, fat-binding, and dough-forming agents. It is uncommon for American women to seek out and purchase foods specifically because they contain soybeans. But, as you will see, it is not that difficult to include more soy products in your diet.

Researchers at the National Institute of Environmental Health Sciences recently conducted a study in which postmenopausal women were fed a variety of soybean-based foods for two months. The women ate a main dish every day containing the equivalent of about one-half cup of soybeans, as well as two soy snacks. The daily snacks consisted of about two ounces of either roasted soy nuts or a cracker spread. The authors of the study estimated that each woman consumed over two hundred milligrams of isoflavones *each day* throughout the two-month period. We can conclude from this study that it is indeed possible for you to get a plentiful amount of soy isoflavones from foods you eat.

Several researchers believe that isoflavones are capable of blocking estrogen's dangerous actions in breast cells, thereby reducing cell growth. Less growth lowers a woman's chances for hazardous DNA mutations within her breast cells. This fact could translate into a possible decrease in a woman's risk for a malignant tumor.

Another interesting fact about soybeans: One particular isoflavone, called *genistein*, acts in at least three other ways to reduce the growth of breast cells. Genistein inhibits two key enzyme pathways that may take part in tumor-growth processes. A recent 1993 report has demonstrated that this soybean isoflavone is even capable of limiting the blood supply to tumors, further reducing abnormal cell growth.

We have several reasons, therefore, to believe that greater consumption of soybean-derived phytochemicals, particularly isoflavones, can play a crucial role in breast cancer protection. You can put this information to work *at once*. Consider the amount of isoflavones in the following soybean products.

Product	Isoflavone Content	Typical Amount Used	Total
Soy sauce	Absent	½–1 teaspoon	0
Soy chips or nuts	1.4 milligram/gram	1 ounce (30 grams)	42
Soy flour	0.4–0.5 milligram/gram	100 grams	50
Tofu	0.5–1 milligram/gram	4 ounces (120 grams)	80
Soy milk	6 milligram/ounce	6–8 ounces	50

The more common soy-based foods eaten in China, Thailand, Korea, Japan, and so on, include tofu (a solid cheeselike product), soy milk, miso and tempeh (both fermented soybean products), soy flour, soy-protein isolate, and soy sauce. Some of these may sound strange to American ears, but they have been staples of the Asian diet for well over two thousand years.

The soybean is surprisingly adaptable and nutritionally complete. Soy protein, an economical, nourishing low-fat vegetable product, forms a major part of vegetarian burgers, which are being tested by the major international fast-food chains.

Canned or packaged soy milk has been available in the United States for many years, although its taste in the past was usually as bland as that of powdered skim milk. Due to the growing demand for healthier food products, however, several newer companies are distributing a wider variety of flavors. Soy milk can be blended with such ingredients as fresh berries or other fresh fruits, maple syrup, vanilla extract, fruit juices, or honey to make delicious cold fruit shakes.

But the soybean product found most often in the refrigerator case in your local supermarket is probably tofu. This soft white block resembles a piece of fresh cheese. The amazing thing about tofu is that, although it has a bland taste on its own, it can readily be turned into main dishes, side dishes, dips, spreads, and great-tasting desserts. Tofu has the remarkable quality of assuming whatever flavor you add to it, whether it's used in stir-fried vegetables, sautéed chicken pieces, with fresh fruits, or to create "cheesecake," enchiladas, or tofu almandine.

Despite its remarkable nutritional properties, tofu has usually been relegated in the United States to Asian households, Chinese restaurants, and vegetarians. Yet earlier in this century, according to John Paino, cofounder of Nasoya, Inc., a U.S. manufacturer of soy-based products, the famous carmaker Henry Ford became such a strong advocate of soy products that he even wore a suit made entirely of soybean fibers.

"Don't cut out tacos, chili, lasagna, pizza, and other treats, simply deliciously remake them with tofu," writes Paino, coauthor with Lisa Messinger of *The Tofu Book*. When you begin to use it, you will discover tofu comes in various textures, from silken (ultrasmooth) to firm to extrafirm. Soybeans are even available in the ice cream alternative Tofutti.

Nutritionally, soybeans are like other legumes (such as peanuts), some of which contain a fairly large amount of vegetable oil. Most of the oil in soybeans is unsaturated, and all of it is cholesterol-free. A four-ounce serving of tofu compares favorably to a typical four-ounce serving of London broil (sliced steak), as shown below.

	4 Oz. of Tofu	4 Oz. of Steak
Protein (g)	11	20
Total fat (g)	6	16
Saturated fat (g)	below 1	6
Cholesterol (mg)	0	109
Calcium (mg)	130	7
Total calories	94	277
Phytochemicals	abundant	absent

This side-by-side comparison says it all. Attempts to fit tofu into recipes are well worth the effort. Feel free to adapt tofu recipes as you see fit. At first, some dishes may seem to include simply too much tofu. You can feel free to reduce the amount without lowering the overall nutritional value of the recipe. Several suggested recipes are offered in Chapter 13.

The Health Effects of Carotenoids

Carotenoids are a huge family of closely related chemicals, nearly all of which are found exclusively in plants. One carotenoid, beta-carotene, is so similar to vitamin A in its chemical structure that it is regularly converted within our bodies into this vitamin.

In 1993, researchers announced that carotenoids appeared to be linked to the prevention of breast cancer. They found that women with the highest levels of total vitamin A intake had an approximately *20 percent reduction in their rates of breast malignancies*, compared with women with the lowest intake.

Protection did not seem to come from vitamin A supplement pills, however, but from eating the whole foods that contained abundant amounts of vitamin A and other carotenoid compounds. Since large doses of vitamin A in supplement form can be harmful, the amounts of this vitamin taken as a supplement should be carefully limited. The human body seems to have little difficulty with large amounts of carotenoids in foods, particularly beta-carotene. Therefore, eating a wide variety of carotenoid-rich plant foods will be both safe and good for the health of your breasts' cells. Abundant amounts of these amazing natural phytochemicals are available to anyone who eats a diet high in fruits and vegetables.

Which vegetables and fruits are rich in carotenoid compounds? The answer is presented in the table on page 113. You will notice the vitamin A content of a particular food is expressed in terms of retinol equivalents, or RE. You will occasionally find vitamin A levels expressed in terms of international units, or IU. The recommended daily allowance (RDA) for vitamin A is 800 RE (equals 4,000 IU). It is recommended that women and men do not exceed 10,000 RE of vitamin A each day.

Foods rich in vitamin A will invariably contain large amounts of dozens of other carotenoids as well, compounds such as lutein, lycopene, alpha-carotene, and cryptoxanthin. As you can see, some foods such as carrots, sweet potatoes, and pumpkin are veritable storehouses of carotenoids.

Vitamin A and other carotenoids have beneficial effects on all cells of our bodies, including breast cells. Their helpful effects, however, do not appear to involve the hormone estrogen. Instead, these phytochemicals protect women by guarding the cells' DNA against activated oxygen (also called free radicals). Vitamin A–like compounds encourage cells in the body to grow in an orderly manner, thereby helping those cells to avoid becoming cancerous. They counteract the effects of cancer-causing genes, called oncogenes.

Several of the vegetables rich in carotenoids are also crucifers— for example, Chinese cabbage, kale, collards, and turnip greens. This may help to explain why vegetable foods work in so many ways to improve our health. Carotenoids clearly exert several healthful effects on the cells of the body, including breast cells. We can conclude that a breast-healthy diet should contain plentiful amounts of natural vitamin A–like substances.

Fiber's Effects on Intestinal Estrogen

In recent years, dietary fiber has come to be seen as an important component of a healthy diet, and rightly so. The term *fiber* includes many things. The simplest definition, however, is that fiber is the portion of the plant that cannot be directly digested by our bodies. The National Cancer Institute believes that most of us eat far less than the recommended twenty-five to thirty-five grams of fiber each day.

There are two principal types of fiber: *soluble* and *insoluble*. Soluble fiber includes such things as gums (guar gum, locust bean gum, xanthan gum), agar, and pectins, all of which are currently being put to good use in manufacturing novel low-fat foods. Even though

RICH NATURAL SOURCES OF VITAMIN A
AND OTHER CAROTENOIDS

VEGETABLES	SERVING SIZE	AMOUNT OF VITAMIN A (RE)
Beet greens	½ cup	734
Chinese cabbage	½ cup, boiled	436
Carrots	1 medium	4,050
Swiss chard	½ cup, chopped	552
Chicory greens	½ cup	720
Collards	½ cup	1,016
Dandelion greens	½ cup, chopped	784
Garden cress	½ cup	1,048
Kale	½ cup	962
Mustard greens	½ cup	670
New Zealand spinach	½ cup, boiled	652
Pumpkin, canned	½ cup	5,380
Seaweed	3.5 ounces	1,040
Spinach	½ cup, boiled	1,474
Sweet potato	1 medium	4,976
Tomato	1 medium	278
Turnip greens	½ cup, boiled	792
Winter squash	½ cup, mashed	1,232
FRUITS		
Apricots, dried	10 halves	2,530
Cantaloupe	1 cup pieces	5,160
Mango	1 medium	8,060
Papaya	1 medium	6,120
Persimmon	1 medium	3,640
Peaches, dried	10 halves	2,810
Prunes	10 dried	1,670

we may not be able to digest these soluble fibers, our intestinal bacteria can. In other words, these soluble fibers do not merely pass through the intestines unchanged. The other major type is insoluble fiber; it includes the cellulose-rich parts of whole wheat and other grains. Wheat bran and whole-wheat breads are some of the best sources of insoluble fiber.

Soluble and insoluble fibers are distinct from one another in some key ways. For example, soluble fiber can be digested by intestinal bacteria, while insoluble fiber cannot. Soluble fiber tends to alter the acidity of the intestinal contents, whereas insoluble fiber doesn't. Each plant food has its own characteristic fiber profile. Because of these differences, each fiber-rich food has its own unique effect on the body.

There is an important link between the dietary fiber a woman eats and the estrogen in her body. After estrogen hormones have done their necessary work in the breasts and other cells, they must be properly eliminated. If not, estrogen would continue to accumulate in the body and might eventually reach dangerously high levels. It is the function of the intestines and the kidneys to dispose of excessive estrogen.

Women are often surprised to learn they normally excrete a large percentage of the body's estrogen each day in their bowel movements. These *intestinal estrogens* are sent from the liver into the intestines as part of the bile and then eliminated. However, the contents of the intestines may take up to twenty-four hours (or more) to pass through the body. There is plenty of time, therefore, for a significant proportion of the intestinal estrogen to be reabsorbed *back into the body*. This reabsorption of estrogen from the intestines is greatly affected by the amount of fiber you eat each day.

Because a certain amount of intestinal estrogen returns directly to the bloodstream, it, too, constitutes a part of the Estrogen Pathway. Intestinal estrogens are, therefore, included as a part of step two, the circulation of estrogen throughout the body.

We know breast cells need estrogen to grow. The more estrogen, the more growth. And the more growth, the greater the risk for cancerous mutations. If greater amounts of intestinal estrogen are being eliminated with the body's wastes, there will be less risk to the breasts. This is precisely why a high-fiber diet seems to be useful for women.

Scientists at the Tufts–New England Medical Center in Boston were among the first to focus attention on this important relationship among fiber, intestinal estrogen, and breast cancer. In a fascinating series of experiments, these researchers were able to show the more a woman's bowel movements weighed each day (due mostly to eating more fiber), the lower her body's estrogen levels.

Other researchers have confirmed the important relationship between stool fiber content and lower estrogen levels in a woman's body. A recent study, for example, looked at sixty-two young women who doubled their daily fiber intake during a two-month period by eating foods fortified with either wheat, rice, or corn bran. The scientists found that estrogen levels were substantially reduced *only* when women were eating the additional wheat bran. This finding made sense because wheat bran is composed mostly of cellulose (an insoluble fiber), and cellulose has been found in test-tube experiments to attach tightly to estrogens.

Scientists have, therefore, come to recognize three basic mechanisms by which dietary fiber might benefit breast cancer risk. First, greater amounts of all fiber make the intestinal contents heavier, trapping more estrogen inside as the stool moves out of the body. Second, some types of insoluble fiber, such as wheat bran, stick tightly to the estrogen they encounter in the intestines, thus aiding the intestinal elimination of the hormone. Third, some fruit and vegetable phytochemicals, called glucarates, actually prevent intestinal estrogen from returning to a woman's bloodstream.

By eating larger amounts of cereal grains, fresh fruits, and vegetables, you can be sure all three intestinal mechanisms contribute to helping the accumulated estrogen pass silently out of your body, minimizing the breast's risks for harmful stimulation.

SOME EXAMPLES OF FIBER-RICH FOODS

Food Item	Total Grams of Fiber
Kellogg Raisin Bran (¾ cup)	5.0
Arnold Bran'nola Original Bread (2 slices)	6.0
Spinach pasta (one cup)	5.2
Weight Watchers Chicken Divan Potato	8.0
Lean Cuisine Zucchini Lasagna	5.3
Pritikin Navy Bean Soup (10 oz. can)	11.0
Health Valley Lentil Soup	5.9
Baked potato with skin (large)	4.2
Corn, cooked (½ cup)	3.1
Figs, dried (3)	5.3
Apple with skin (large), or pear	4.7
Orange (medium)	3.1
Popcorn, air-popped (3 cups)	3.9
Pinto beans (¾ cup cooked beans)	14.2

Bioflavonoids and Other New Directions in Phytochemical Research

The term *bioflavonoid*, refers to a very large group of chemicals found throughout the plant world. Members of this chemical family are present in every plant we eat. It has been estimated that anyone who eats even a few servings of fruits and vegetables will consume *one thousand to two thousand milligrams* of these compounds each day. Naturally, vegetarians consume much more than this amount.

Nearly sixty years ago, Dr. Albert Szent-Györgyi, the Nobel Prize–winning biochemist who helped discover vitamin C, gave bioflavonoids the name "vitamin P." He had noticed these plant chemicals were excellent antioxidants and that they seemed to prevent scurvy, just like vitamin C. He concluded that bioflavonoids must also be vitamins, probably essential to human health. Though the concept of "vitamin P" has not stood the test of time and has been abandoned, it is clear bioflavonoids are beneficial to our health.

Bioflavonoids occur in many different chemical forms. It is not surprising to find that some of them have effects on biochemical pathways in humans. Medical scientists have shown that some bioflavonoids are able to inhibit the key enzymes that produce estrogen. By limiting the production of estrogen, these plant chemicals interfere with step one of the Estrogen Pathway.

Other researchers have found that several of the common bioflavonoids in one's diet can increase the production of protective enzymes in the tissues. These enzymes act by detoxifying certain substances you might find in your food, such as pesticides. This fact helps to explain why diets rich in plant foods are so protective against cancers in humans. The detoxifying pathways in our bodies also help to reduce the excessive activity of estrogen, both by producing more inactive C-2 estrogen and by speeding the removal of these hormones from our bodies.

Like most phytochemical research, the investigation of the role of bioflavonoids in human health is in its infancy. Much more work needs to be done to identify how much of which bioflavonoid may be most advantageous to breast health. Since bioflavonoids are present in *all* fruits and vegetables, you can assure yourself of an abundant supply by eating a wide variety of these wonderful plant foods.

We have focused here on just a few groups of phytochemicals important to breast health, those for which a considerable amount of scientific evidence already exists. Our study of the enormous plant world and its amazing pharmaceutical-like substances has a long way to go. New research leads are coming in from several directions. Consider, for example, just two new plant substances emerging on the breast cancer prevention scene: *limonene* and *lignans*.

Limonene is present in citrus fruits, such as oranges, lemons, limes, kumquats, grapefruit, and citron. It has been found actually to reverse the course of breast tumors in experimental animals.

Lignans share some of the properties of the isoflavones, and scientists have observed reduced breast tumors in experimental animals consuming plants that contain them. Lignans are found predominantly in whole grains, including flax seed and whole-rye grain, as well as in various beans.

Each of these phytochemicals, along with dozens of others, are undergoing intense study in laboratories all over the world. As this exciting work continues, a clearer picture of the potential role of these phytochemical agents in cancer prevention will undoubtedly emerge.

In time, it may even prove possible to create food products enriched with specific phytochemicals. Medical research, however, is expensive and time-consuming. If women are to benefit *soon* from such products, a greater investment in research from the food industry, as well as from governmental and private sources, will be necessary.

The food industry, furthermore, will have to exercise greater discipline if such innovative food products are ever to come to market. Only in this way will food manufacturers win the trust and participation of researchers, for whom even a hint of advertising hype can result in the permanent loss of scientific credibility. The consumer needs to be wary of extravagant health claims made for any food product. Some companies, sad to say, may be concerned more with the health of their profits than with the health of the people who purchase their goods. It will take a new spirit of trust and cooperation among government, industry, and the academic research community to design and test these new products.

In the next chapter, we will see exactly how you can begin to alter your diet to include at least five servings *per day* of the powerful breast cancer-fighting phytochemicals we have discussed here.

WHAT DIETARY CHANGES MUST YOU MAKE NOW?

As we showed you earlier, your diet is the cornerstone to a comprehensive strategy for reducing breast cancer risk. No other approach
meets all of these five criteria: *The recommended changes are under
your control. The changes are both simple and enjoyable. Change can
begin today. The changes will protect you from other cancers and chronic
diseases in addition to breast cancer. These dietary changes can protect
your entire family.* In this chapter and the next, we will discuss
dietary strategies aimed primarily at reducing *your* risk for breast
cancer. Some of them will undoubtedly sound familiar and seem
relatively simple.

Current Official Nutritional Guidelines

There is a broad scientific consensus about the dietary changes we
all need to make to reduce our cancer risk. The recommendations
listed below are essentially those offered by the American Cancer

Society, the U.S. National Cancer Institute, the U.S. National Research Council, and the U.S. Preventive Services Task Force:

1. Avoid obesity. In order to achieve and maintain your proper body weight, limit your daily calorie intake and exercise aerobically on a routine basis for at least thirty minutes three to four times per week.
2. Reduce total fat intake to no more than 30 percent of your total daily calories. Limit your intake of saturated fat by reducing consumption of meats, eggs, cheeses, and other animal products.
3. Include at least five servings of a variety of fresh fruits and green and yellow vegetables in your daily diet (the Five-a-Day for Better Health program).
4. Consume more high-fiber foods, such as whole-grain products, legumes (beans), and fruits and vegetables. Total fiber intake should not exceed thirty-five grams per day.
5. If you consume alcoholic beverages, limit yourself to two drinks daily (as defined by five ounces of wine, twelve ounces of beer, or about one and a half ounces of vodka, whiskey, or similar liquor).
6. Minimize your consumption of smoked, salt-cured, and nitrite-cured foods.

Other well-respected organizations, however, insist that *some of these national recommendations do not go far enough.* The Center for Science in the Public Interest (CSPI), a Washington, D.C.–based activist group and publisher of *The Nutrition Action Health Letter,* in an article entitled, "Ho-Hum Diet Advice" (May 1989), criticized the thirteen-hundred-page 1989 report of the U.S. National Research Council, arguing that changes like the ones listed above are merely those that fit most conveniently into American lifestyles.

The CSPI article points out that many of the authors of this huge report have acknowledged elsewhere that *eating even less total and saturated fat, cholesterol, and sodium than they recommended would lead to better health.* "But," CSPI contends, "they lacked the courage to tell the public *how much less.* In doing so, they passed up a terrific chance to offer us their vision of what the optimal diet should look like."

We strongly believe women should try to limit their fat consumption to *20 percent or less* of total daily calorie intake. Only a level of fat intake well below 30 percent of daily calories appears to reduce estrogen in your body, as demonstrated among the participants in the Women's Health Trial. Lowering total fat consumption also reduces the potential harm to your body from saturated fats.

The goal of a 20 percent fat diet can be achieved by focusing more attention each day on vegetables, fruits, breads, cereals, and pasta. With a little effort, fat can be successfully removed from most of the foods you eat, with little sacrifice of taste or enjoyment.

As a general rule, women must also reduce their dependence on meat and whole-milk dairy products as a primary source of protein. Other excellent sources of protein can be found in whole grains and beans, especially soybeans. When choosing dairy products, use low-fat or skim-milk products, including low-fat cheeses.

Choose lean cuts of beef, fish, or skinless white-meat chicken or turkey, and limit the portions by serving these meats with more vegetables. Most Asian women are not vegetarians; they simply do not rely on meat products to make up the major food item in their recipes, as we tend to do.

With these broad principles in mind, let's examine some of the specific strategies useful in creating your own breast-healthy diet.

For Your Eyes Only

Before considering any dietary strategy, you will first need to complete a seven-day food diary. Whether you are young or old, there is no more useful dietary learning tool than a personal food diary. Although you will not be able to analyze this record as a nutritionist might, a food diary can be an invaluable tool for showing you *exactly* what you are eating at this time in your life. It will be especially valuable for comparison purposes in the future.

The first step in preparing a food diary is very simple: Take at least seven pieces of three-hole lined schoolbook paper and staple them together. Now write the name of the days of the week across the top of each page. Find a way to keep this invaluable packet with you at all times over the next week.

Step two is just as easy. *Write down everything you eat—from Sunday morning to the following Saturday night.* Write down everything—and we mean exactly that—*everything.* Go for details. If you like two teaspoons of sugar in your coffee, write it down. Do you always have a doughnut, a bag of pretzels, or crumb cake with your coffee break? Write it down. Make notes in your diary about the times you eat these things.

A few pistachios offered by a friend? A box of M&M's on the way home from work? A glass of wine? Write it down. This cannot be overemphasized. *Everything* in the way of food or drink that enters your mouth must be included on your seven-day food diary, with the possible exception of water. Remember: It's for your eyes only. You must avoid altering your daily eating habits simply because you are paying close attention to them. Nobody needs to see this food diary but you. Therefore, be perfectly honest with yourself. Write down everything you eat during these seven days.

If you pay attention to details, it will help you to learn what you need to know about the foods you currently eat. How large exactly was that serving of meat last night? Four ounces (about the size of a deck of cards), or more? How was the meat prepared? Was there a sauce? How was it prepared? Learn to estimate the correct serving sizes of the foods you eat. A measuring cup equals eight ounces, and a pint of cottage cheese or sour cream is two cups, or sixteen ounces.

Admittedly, a seven-day food diary can be a tedious and time-consuming task. Yet all dietary recommendations are linked to it. It is certainly worth your time and effort. Once it's finished, *date it*, then save it. Let's summarize some of the benefits to you from completing a seven-day food diary:

1. *You will learn about the importance of serving sizes.*
   This is extremely important—it will help in calculating how many calories or fat/fiber grams you eat each day.

2. *You will learn when you are most vulnerable to overeating or snacking.*
   Most of us do not realize that there are certain patterns to the way we eat each day. A daily food diary will reveal that to you.
3. *You will begin to pay closer attention to the composition of foods.*
   It is essential that you become aware of what goes into making up a particular food or recipe. This will be important when you try to improve your diet.
4. *You will become aware of what you are not eating.*
   Your food diary will help you determine whether or not you are eating your average of five to nine servings of fruits and vegetables each day.
5. *You will be able to compare your current eating habits with your diet in the future.*
   This is perhaps the most gratifying reason of all, since you will have permanent proof of the valuable changes you have made in your approach to food and health.

Obstacles to Dietary Change: Our Fast-Food/ Fat-Food Culture

"Fast food as big business," writes Lila Perl in *Junk Food, Fast Food, Health Food*, "is a phenomenon of 20th century America that began to zoom during the 1950's." The social and economic changes of the postwar decades created enormous opportunities for the growth of the fast-food industry. The busier and more hectic our lives became, the more the advertising slogans reassured us that we really did "deserve a break today" and tomorrow and every day.

Fast food, we are constantly told, is fun, exciting, and satisfying. Unfortunately, fast food is often fat food. Fat is important to the food industry for two reasons. First, the high proportion of fat in such foods is a cheap and easy way to add flavor to otherwise-bland mass-produced products. Second, fat is rich in calories, so customers will invariably feel full. Just how much fat is in some of these fast foods? Take a look at the following table.

TOTAL GRAMS OF FAT IN SINGLE SERVINGS OF COMMON FAST FOODS

MISCELLANEOUS FAST-FOOD ITEMS*		POPULAR ITEMS AT McDONALD'S†	
Mexican Pizza at Taco Bell	37 grams	Quarter Pounder w/Cheese	28 grams
Jr. Swiss Deluxe at Wendy's	18	Quarter Pounder	20
Chicken Sandwich at KFC	27	Cheeseburger	13
Hamburger Deluxe at Wendy's	21	Big Mac	26
Cheeseburger at Burger King	15	Filet-O-Fish	18
Burrito Supreme at Taco Bell	22	McChicken	20
Cheese Pan Pizza at Pizza Hut	18	Large French Fries	22
Big Deluxe at Hardees	30	Egg McMuffin	11
Bacon Cheeseburger at Hardees	39	Sausage Biscuit with Egg	33
Taco Salad/with Shell at Taco Bell	61	Iced Cheese Danish	21
Popcorn Chicken at KFC	45	Choclaty Chip Cookies	15

*Source: Center for Science in the Public Interest

†Source: *McDonald's Nutrition and You—A Guide to Healthy Eating at McDonald's*, 1991, McDonald's Corp.

A simple calculation will help you to realize how much fat this really is. Suppose that a woman weighs 130 pounds and needs to eat about sixteen hundred calories a day. By setting a limit of 20 percent of calories from fat, she should not be eating more than thirty-six grams of fat daily. Think about this for a moment—a lunchtime Quarter Pounder with cheese and french fries has exceeded this individual's allowable fat intake for the entire day.

The following table shows the grams of fat women eat on various diets.

ESTIMATING GRAMS OF FAT ALLOWED EACH DAY ON VARIOUS DIETS

BODY WEIGHT	DAILY CALORIES	GRAMS OF FAT ALLOWED			
(lb.)		20% Fat Diet	25% Fat Diet	30% Fat Diet	40% Fat Diet
100	1,200	27	33	40	53
110	1,300	29	36	43	58
120	1,400	31	39	47	62
130	1,600	36	44	53	71
140	1,700	38	47	56	76
150	1,800	40	50	60	80
160	1,900	42	52	63	84
170	2,000	44	56	67	89
180	2,200	49	61	73	98

Trying to avoid the hidden fat in the American diet can seem like trying to cross a field of land mines without a detector. Product advertising can be deceptive. You may have no idea just how fatty some products really are. While new food labels soon to be required by the FDA should make it easier to find the fat hidden in the foods we eat, fat will undoubtedly continue to be a major component of many processed foods. Just consider the fat content of some items we found in a local supermarket.

Mrs. Paul's Deviled Crabs: eighteen grams of fat for only two crab cakes.

Gorton's Crunchy Battered Fish Sticks: nineteen grams of fat in two fish sticks.

Pepperidge Farm Vegetables in Pastry—Broccoli with Cheese: sixteen grams of fat per serving.

Sanwa Foods Ramen Soup: sixteen grams of fat per serving.

Kraft Macaroni & Cheese: thirteen grams of fat per three-quarters of a cup.

Celeste Pepperoni Pizza: 26.1 grams of fat per one-third of a pie.

Sara Lee Banana Nut Bran Muffin: eighteen grams of fat per muffin.

Sara Lee Golden Corn Muffin: fourteen grams of fat per muffin.

Eggo Homestyle Waffle: ten grams of fat per two waffles.

Contadina Alfredo Pasta Sauce: thirty-four grams of fat per four ounces.

In addition to fast foods, the convenience of dining out also has considerable time-saving appeal to many women and their families. Restaurant meals will contribute to your overall consumption of hidden fat calories. Diners have little control over what goes into preparing the foods in a restaurant. And you can be certain that the restaurant owner will generally select high-fat recipes to appeal to the expectations of most of his customers.

What do people usually order in a restaurant? The more popular food items served to young women and men are the following: buffalo chicken wings; fried mozzarella sticks; fried calamari; potato skins filled with bacon and cheese; nachos; pepperoni pizza; and tacos filled with ground meat, cheese, and sour cream. Each of these items is bursting at the seams with fat calories! Yet many customers believe the fat is what makes the items seem so delicious and filling. There is simply no motivation whatsoever to remove or limit the fat in most restaurant foods.

Fast foods are not the only problem interfering with a healthy low-fat diet. Fat is a major ingredient of most snack foods as well, adding that certain taste we have been conditioned to expect. Once you start to nibble, it's difficult to stop. After all, do you know *anyone* who can get by on just one potato or corn chip? In fact, eating snack foods is a preference many of us learn early in life and continue throughout adulthood. It is this lifelong allegiance that snack-food manufacturers cultivate.

What about the food value of these snack foods? Most of these products contain nine to ten grams of fat *per ounce*. Since many people eating these snack foods will easily (and quickly) consume two to four ounces, this can add up to a whopping amount of fat. This is a serious problem, particularly for children, since these salty, calorie-dense foods quickly fill the child, leaving him or her with little further appetite.

In the end, as much as one-third of the total calories eaten by some women comes from foods with very little nutritional benefit: sodas, (salty) snacks, wine, cookies, doughnuts, and candy. By relying on fatty fast foods and soft drinks, a woman's eating pattern can easily become lopsided. It can become top-heavy with fats and simple sugars and too light in fruits, vegetables, fruit and vegetable juices, whole grains, and low-fat dairy products.

Given our national pattern of fat consumption, it isn't at all surprising that fat calories have been viewed as the greatest hazard to breast cells. Many of these extremely fatty foods appeared in our food supply just as breast cancer rates began to rise dramatically throughout the 1960s and 1970s.

Personal strategies to limit overall fat intake, combined with increased fruit and vegetable consumption, will require that women overcome all of these obstacles associated with our fast-food/fat-food culture. Let us, therefore, turn our attention to seven specific dietary steps that you can begin *today*.

CHAPTER TEN.

SEVEN DIETARY STRATEGIES

The actual changes you will need to make in your eating habits to achieve a breast-healthy diet are surprisingly few. The strategies for realizing this goal are simple to understand and implement. They can be summarized as follows:

1. Introduce new dietary changes *slowly*.
2. Consume *more* fruits and vegetables.
3. *Try* new recipes.
4. Know *what's* in the foods you eat.
5. *Total* it up: Keep track of what you eat.
6. Obtain the correct amount of dietary *fiber*.
7. Find *substitutes* for fattier foods.

Strategy Number 1: Introduce New Dietary Changes *Slowly*

The first guideline for ensuring lasting dietary changes is to keep things simple and to *make changes slowly*. Because most of our eating habits have been acquired over an entire lifetime, they cannot be unlearned overnight. While some might argue our culture's "fat tooth" is attributable to the rich, "wonderful" taste and flavor of fatty foods, in fact much of this is merely a habit. Most of us have grown up on fast foods, chips, doughnuts, and soft drinks. These dietary preferences can be unlearned, but it takes time to make gradual changes in the way you eat and *to stick to them*. We are not talking about a diet that you go on, merely to go off again.

Participants in the Women's Health Trial soon came to enjoy and favor low-fat food choices, even to the point where the taste of fatty foods became disagreeable to them. Again, for those women, the process took place *slowly*, over at least one year for most, and even longer for others. This process of dietary adjustment is similar to the experience of adding less salt to your food or less sugar to your coffee. You will certainly notice the difference at first and may even dislike it. But eventually, you will view the new taste as "normal." Indeed, while you may crave the old-fashioned tastes of fattier foods as they are gradually eliminated, this craving will not last for long, and it is more than balanced by a slimmer and healthier you.

Most physicians and researchers agree that changes made slowly have the best chance of becoming permanently integrated into a person's lifestyle. For example, it does you and your family little good to eliminate *all* cream, butter, or cheese from a recipe if you aren't ready for the change. It may be too much of a culinary shock. If the total elimination of certain foods in your diet is viewed emotionally as a punishment, you may experience what some behavioral scientists call "aversive conditioning." This is actually the best way to train someone *not* to do something!

How do you start to make healthier food choices? The answer is by taking lots of little steps. Introduce *small amounts* of newer kinds of vegetables into soups, stews, salads, or stir-fry recipes. Add *small cubes of tofu* to your stir-fry recipes, along with slightly smaller portions of beef or chicken. Within a few months, you and your family will become accustomed to these important sources of nutrients and cancer-fighting phytochemicals. And once you have become more familiar with these new tastes, you can gradually increase the amounts eaten at one time.

Strategy Number 2: Consume *More* Fruits and Vegetables

This message has been the leading theme of our book. According to recommendations of the National Cancer Institute, each woman should strive to eat *at least* five—and, better yet, nine—servings of fruits and vegetables *each day*. As many women have discovered, you can eat *more* of these protective foods without necessarily gaining more pounds.

What, then, is a serving? Let us review what the experts recommend, based on the average amount normally eaten at a time. A serving of fruits or vegetables consists of one of the following:

- one medium-sized piece of fresh fruit
- three-quarters of a cup, or six ounces, of 100 percent fruit juice (for example, tomato juice or orange juice)
- one cup of uncooked leafy vegetables
- one-half a cup of cooked or raw vegetables
- one-half a cup of diced or cooked fruit
- one-quarter of a cup of dried fruit

Here are some suggested ways you might achieve the five to nine servings you should be eating each day. Realize that each of the servings of fruits and vegetables suggested here are rich in their own unique complement of phytochemicals. All of these foods have the *potential* to reduce breast cancer risk, although, as we have seen, some plant foods seem to be much more effective than others.

Breakfast: A serving would include any of the following: a cup of orange juice, one-half a cup of sliced bananas, strawberries, or blueberries on your cereal, a few dried apricots or raisins (about two ounces), half a grapefruit or some other piece of fruit.

If you are accustomed to running out the door without eating breakfast, it is very important to try gradually to eliminate this habit. Studies have repeatedly shown that people who skip breakfast usually make up for their missed calories later in the day by eating high-fat snack foods. In addition, it becomes much more difficult to fit in the five to nine servings of fruits and vegetables each day if you don't start eating until a midmorning coffee break or later.

Snack (at any time during the day): A serving here could be a piece of fruit—for example, a small bunch of grapes, an apple, pear, orange, or a tangerine. Try taking a little box of raisins or a four-once bag of carrot sticks with you to work. Each qualifies as a serving. Also, how about doubling up sometime? Have an orange *and* an apple if you're in the mood. There are only a few added calories from such a choice, unlike when you eat two doughnuts or two slices of pizza.

Lunch: Drink a small can of Campbell's V-8 juice with lunch, an individual carton of pink grapefruit juice, or 100 percent apple juice. Bring along a sliced tomato. If you weren't in the mood for fruit as an earlier snack, have one or two servings for lunch. Try some dried dates, figs, or dried apricots. In the summertime, you can choose from an abundance of ripe cherries, strawberries, melon slices, juicy plums, or peaches.

Even eating lunch out provides an opportunity to get one or two servings of fruits and vegetables, providing you choose wisely. Enjoy the salad bar or have a potato baked in the skin. But remember, at a salad bar it is wise to avoid the bacon bits and fried croutons, as well as the creamy dressings. Salads and baked potatoes do not have to be drowned in fat to taste good.

Dinner: This is an excellent time to add to your fresh fruit and vegetable quota. *Routinely* have a green salad or coleslaw with your meals. Mix in an assortment of raw vegetables, such as sliced red radishes, cherry tomatoes, cucumber slices, strips of red, green, or yellow peppers. Do what Italians enjoy doing: Mix a wide assortment of different leafy green vegetables in your salad, such as chicory, watercress, endive, and red-leaf lettuce. Toss in some chopped parsley or fragrant fresh dill and serve this salad with a low-fat or nonfat spicy dressing.

You can serve several hot vegetables at the dinner table, in combination if you wish. For example, try zucchini *and* corn niblets mixed with stewed tomatoes and a sprinkling of basil or oregano. What about a delicious cabbage-vegetable soup? You will find several easy-to-prepare recipes in this book. Serve a baked or microwaved potato, or, better yet, use vitamin A-rich sweet potatoes instead. Sweet potatoes are terrific when mashed with either applesauce or orange juice and a little brown sugar instead of butter or margarine. You will find it is possible to add a variety of nonfat spices, herbs, sauces, and condiments to enhance the flavor of vegetables.

Desserts: Here is another good opportunity to add some fresh fruit to your nonfat frozen yogurt or refreshing sorbet. Top it with fresh sliced peaches, strawberries, blueberries, or raspberries. You can cut up any combination of fresh fruit and mix it with a little fruit juice and a dash of sweet wine or a cordial. Make the fruit salad at least a half hour in advance, if possible, and let the juice and the wine combine into a delicious sauce.

Juicing: As a result of widespread and aggressive TV advertising, juicers have found their way into the kitchens of thousands of American women. It is difficult for any of us to ignore the enthusiasm of a television salesperson as he or she announces the incredible health benefits of this or that vegetable juice. However, as we saw in the previous two chapters, the phytochemical contents of a particular fruit or vegetable are not limited to its juice.

Moreover, some important vegetables, like cabbage or broccoli, have very little juice at all. We have learned how the soluble and insoluble fibers in these plant foods play an important role in safely helping to eliminate intestinal estrogen in women. You simply don't receive the benefit of these fibers if you use most juicers.

Any attempt to extract *only* the juice from a combination of fruits and/or vegetables will usually result in a considerable *loss* of the nutrient and phytochemical contents. Given the power of plant foods to promote our health, such a loss of fiber and trapped phytochemicals, over a long period of time, can only be detrimental. Obviously, an occasional enjoyment of a flavorful drink containing fresh carrot or apple juice is not the problem. But when the nutritious pulp of these vegetables or fruit is going to waste, *all of the valuable fibers and trapped phytochemicals you would have received* by eating the entire fruit or vegetable are lost to you, as well.

Strategy Number 3: *Try New Recipes*

One of the most important dietary strategies taught to women in the Women's Health Trial was the incorporation of *new* low-fat recipes into their cooking. With a little experimentation, an adventuresome spirit, and some determination, you, too, will discover your ability to cook entirely novel dishes that are both easy to prepare and enjoyable to all.

It has been observed that many of us often prepare and eat the same five or six meals, week in and week out. This statistic tells us that a certain amount of effort will have to be made in order to expand the habitual selections made routinely by most women when they set about preparing a meal.

The first step in discovering and eventually incorporating newer recipes into your lifestyle is to be able to tell the difference between a relatively healthy recipe and one that is not. In general, the more butter, cream, or vegetable oil a recipe calls for, the more likely it is that fats make up the bulk of the total calories. And, as we noted earlier, when fat is plentiful, something else has given way to make room for these calories, usually vegetables.

Most recipe books geared to health-conscious women will explicitly tell you the number of fat grams in a single serving of the dish. Make it a point to look for this information. Naturally, the lower the total fat, the better. You will always notice in low-fat recipes that the author has found a way of using an alternative to oil to make up the sauce, usually choosing instead a low-fat yogurt, low-salt chicken stock, beef bouillon, or wine. Each oil substitute adds its own unique flavor. Therefore, the need for fat in the recipe is eliminated without sacrificing taste.

A desirable or breast-healthy recipe for the purpose of breast cancer prevention should give a prominent place to vegetables, fruits, and grains in the dish and a relatively small role to meat. Each of the recipes included in this book will demonstrate this principle.

The women in the Women's Health Trial met frequently with one another to compare recipes and to share their experiences in cooking various low-fat dishes. While many reading this book will not have immediate access to such a support group, a suitable alternative can be found in the increasing number of books and magazine articles with the specific focus of a healthier low-fat lifestyle. Several magazines are exclusively devoted to cooking delicious low-fat, low-calorie recipes. You might also consider the *Nutrition Action Healthletter* published monthly by the CSPI. A listing of helpful cookbooks and other resources will be found in Chapter 11.

Be forewarned, however, that while newspapers, women's magazines, and even local papers pay lip service to the importance of diet and breast cancer prevention, their food pages often give quite the opposite message. Consider a few of the main ingredients included in a recipe featured recently in the food section of a major newspaper. The recipe describes a side dish containing eggplants and potatoes, which might seem like a good way to get your vegetables.

THE RECIPE INCLUDES	GRAMS OF FAT
4 tablespoons unsalted butter	48.8
¼ cup heavy cream	22.4
¼ cup milk	2.2
3½ tablespoons olive oil	47.2
1 tablespoon sesame oil	13.6
1 tablespoon tahini	8.1
Total Fat	142.3 grams
Fat per Serving	35.6 grams

Each serving of this side dish gives each person nearly thirty-six grams of fat—and that's only if you make sure to divide it into four equal servings. The 36 grams of fat per serving doesn't even take into consideration other fat calories a woman might eat in the main dish or dessert.

Consider, too, a recent newspaper article, entitled "Physician Soothes the Palate." In his office, surrounded by syringes and intravenous medications, the local physician holds up his "gourmet specialties." Among these is pasta with vodka sauce. The recipe includes butter, olive oil, prosciutto, and half-and-half. *Each serving* delivers about twenty-three grams of fat.

While the intent of this article was, no doubt, innocent enough, it nonetheless represents the kind of mixed message our society gives about health and nutrition. It is just this sort of contradictory message women need to recognize and screen out.

As an even more ironic example of this problem, we cite the following gourmet recipes for busy women offered by a national women's magazine that is recognized for its commitment to the cause of women's breast health. Here are a few examples:

- Turkey piccata for two: contains one tablespoon of olive oil and four tablespoons of butter or margarine—about twenty-nine grams of fat per serving.
- Eggs Benedict with hollandaise sauce for four: contains one full cup of softened margarine and fourteen egg yolks—about sixty grams of fat per serving.
- Jalapeño quiche for four to six: contains fourteen tablespoons of butter, one cup of sharp cheddar cheese, and one cup of heavy whipping cream—almost seventy-three grams of fat per serving.

The lesson here is simple: Learn to analyze and assess recipes for breast-healthy ingredients and food-preparation methods. Use common sense to evaluate the extent to which a recipe relies upon fats and oils to make it work. *Experiment!* Try recipes aimed at lowering fat and maximizing flavor. You can usually omit or find substitutes for butter, margarine, heavy cream, and high-fat cheeses. By substituting red or white wine, soy sauce (low-sodium), salsa, low-fat dressings, Worcestershire sauce, orange or lemon juice, or Dijon mustard in place of the omitted oils, most recipes can be just as delicious.

The use of fresh herbs such as chopped basil, chives, garlic, parsley, dill, mint, ginger, and cilantro, found in most produce sections, can also add zest and plenty of phytochemicals to foods without adding any fat. Dried spices and herbs such as paprika, garlic, thyme, saffron, pepper, oregano, sage, cinnamon, nutmeg and others can intensify the flavor of a dish. Whenever possible, purchase your spices and herbs in glass containers rather than in the small metal canisters you will find in your supermarket. The bottles can be more tightly closed between uses and will preserve the flavor much longer.

There simply is no need to sacrifice enjoyment for good health. Eating is one of the true pleasures in life. No one wants to feel deprived or eat food that has the flavor of cardboard. Most vegetable-based recipes can be easily altered, for example, if you don't happen to like a particular vegetable or other ingredient. It isn't like baking a cake or pie, where the recipe has to be followed precisely. Consult the listing that follows this chapter for some of the better sources of wonderful low-fat recipes for your enjoyment and health.

Strategy Number 4: Know *What's* in the Foods You Eat

The next tactic is to become very familiar with the ingredients of the foods you eat each day. You simply *must know what is in them.* This is not always easy, however. Consumers will be greatly aided in their efforts to know what is in the foods they eat when the federal food labeling law is fully enacted by May 1994. The new labels will apply to almost all packaged foods, compared with only about 60 percent of food products at present.

This new label was created in response to widespread dissatisfac-

Nutrition Facts

Serving Size 1/2 cup (114g)

Servings Per Container 4

◄

Amount Per Serving

Calories 90   Calories from Fat 30   ◄

% Daily Value*

Total Fat 3g	5% ◄
Saturated Fat 0g	0%
Cholesterol 0mg	0%
Sodium 300mg	13%
Total Carbohydrate 13g	4%
Dietary Fiber 3g	12% ◄
Sugars 3g	
Protein 3g	

Vitamin A	80 %	• Vitamin C	60%
Calcium	4 %	• Iron	4%

*Percent Daily Values are based on a 2,000 calorie diet. Your daily values may be higher or lower depending on your calorie needs:

	Calories	2,000	2,500
Total Fat	Less than	65g	80g
Sat Fat	Less than	20g	25g
Cholesterol	Less than	300mg	300mg
Sodium	Less than	2,400mg	2,400mg
Total Carbohydrate		300g	375g
Fiber		25g	30g

Calories per gram:

Fat 9   •   Carbohydrates 4   •   Protein 4

FIGURE 7

The New FDA Food Label Due to Appear on Most Foods in 1994

tion among consumers, health officials, and nutritionists with the ways foods are now commonly labeled and advertised. Until now, labeling by food manufacturers has been voluntary and not standardized. According to the revised regulations, serving sizes will be meaningful, clearly specified, and uniform for a given line of similar products. Nonspecific terms such as *low, good source, light,* and *free,* long used with almost no guidance, will be restricted.

"The Tower of Babel in food labels has come down, and American consumers are the winners," Dr. Louis W. Sullivan, former secretary of the Department of Health and Human Services, triumphantly proclaimed. Together with Dr. David Kessler, commissioner of the Food and Drug Administration, Dr. Sullivan fought hard for the new rules. They represent, he believes, "a powerful incentive to the food industry to offer healthy food choices." The labeling laws should put an end to some of the confusing and even deceptive practices foisted upon the consumer. No longer, for example, will a company be able to advertise its olive oil as being extralight when it is only the color of the oil that is lighter, not the calorie content.

Many important nutritional gains have been achieved by the labeling laws. The labels themselves, however, may seem too cluttered or too confusing at first. Consumers will have to learn how to use them effectively.

A serious criticism is that the labels have been built around the decision that *30 percent of total calories from fat* is the current best health recommendation for American women. As we have already discussed, women seriously wishing to reduce stimulation to their breasts from estrogen hormones will have to aim lower than 30 percent. The label's lower estimate of two thousand calories per day, apparently meant to include women, allows for up to sixty-five grams of fat each day. This is too many calories and far too much fat for most women. Look again at the daily fat-allowance table found on page 125. The FDA's recommended level of sixty-five grams of fat each day is simply off the scale for many women, particularly those in the lower range of height and weight.

The new labels, moreover, are so filled with food facts, they may appear overwhelming to many of us. We have gone from no information on many products to more information than the average consumer wants to know. Do not be intimidated by all the percentages. The best advice is to zero in on just four factors.

Serving size: Pay close attention to the recommended serving size; it reflects the amounts most people actually eat and it has been made more consistent across various product lines.

Total calories per serving: Total calories add up as soon as you start to eat more than the appropriate serving. For example, the Pepperidge Farm Wholesome Choice Raspberry Tart Cookie contains only one gram of fat and sixty calories each and makes an excellent low-fat snack food. Yet, if you absentmindedly eat several of these cookies, the fat and total calories start to add up.

Total fat: The amount of cholesterol and saturated fat is not as important as the number of *total fat grams* in the food. *Low cholesterol, no cholesterol,* or *low in saturated fats* are advertising buzz terms that will only distract you as you try to select lower-fat foods. Take mayonnaise, for example, made from vegetable oil: over eleven grams of fat per tablespoon, nearly 100 percent of its calories derived from fat, and yet *no cholesterol.*

Dietary fiber: This is one of the key pieces of information on the new food label. As we learned previously, fiber is more than vegetable matter passing undigested through our intestines. It is active in steering excessive estrogen and other dangerous substances safely out of the body. With experience, you will become familiar with a wide variety of enjoyable high-fiber foods.

Strategy Number 5: *Total* It Up: Keep Track of What You Eat

The importance of adding up the total amount of various food components each day should make sense in light of all you have learned about the relationship among food, diet, and breast health.

This is where your training with the food diary will be especially valuable. Pay attention to *what's in the food, what the serving sizes are*, and *how it adds up during the day.*

Fortunately, there are several learning aids to help the average consumer tabulate the fat, fiber, and calorie content of various foods. The Center for Science in the Public Interest has created a handy scorecard called *The Eating Smart Fat Guide,* which tells you at a glance the exact amount of dietary fat and total calories in over two hundred commonly eaten foods. (We will tell you how to obtain this and other helpful resources in the next chapter.)

This clever, fun-to-read four-by-ten-inch guide is small enough to put in your pocket or purse and take to the supermarket. By sliding a card up or down, you line up a particular food and read at the bottom of the card the typical serving size, the total calories, and the total fat grams. The fourteen categories of foods listed include dairy products, cheese and eggs, frozen deserts, fats and oils, cooked fish, grains and cereals, sweet baked goods, crackers and chips, nuts and beans, meats and poultry, frozen and prepared foods listed by brand name, condiments and sauces, sweets, and fast foods.

There may still be several foods you like to eat that are not found on the CSPI fat guide. Most of the necessary information, however, will soon be available on the package label itself. Become an avid reader in the supermarket. Routinely scan the labels on every box, bottle, can, or package you might buy. Some foods you purchase will be approximately the same as those listed on the fat guide. As an additional resource, you may want to buy one of the several fat-gram counters currently available in your bookstore.

Remember: Everything you eat adds up throughout the day, and, eventually, throughout your life. Become familiar with the process of totaling it up, of keeping track of what you eat. You will find you can average out these totals over several different days. For instance, when you feel you want to indulge in an *occasional* ice cream cone or that slice of cake, lower your fat intake over two to three days.

Strategy Number 6: Obtain the Correct Amount of Dietary *Fiber*

When we speak of the "correct" amount of dietary fiber, we are acknowledging that it is possible for someone to get too much fiber. Vitamin and mineral absorption may be adversely affected if you eat more than thirty-five grams of fiber per day. Nevertheless, for most women in America today, the correct amount usually translates into *more fiber*. The average American woman eats barely more than ten grams of fiber each day. Since that number is the average, it tells us that a large number of women consume even fewer than ten grams each day. The current recommendations call for doubling or tripling this number—into the range of at least twenty-five to thirty-five grams of dietary fiber each and every day.

What does it take to consume this amount of fiber each day? To answer this question, it's necessary to identify those foods containing dietary fiber. Luckily, there is CSPI's other easy-to-use scorecard, entitled *The Eating Smart Fiber Guide.* Here, the thirteen categories are cereals; breads; nuts and seeds; cakes, pastries, and muffins; crackers; fast foods; grains and pasta; frozen dinners and entrées; soups; vegetables; fruits and juices; cookies, candies, and chips; and beans, peas, and tofu. Again, simply pull down the center card, line up a food choice from one of these categories, and focus in on the totals. A table of typical fiber-rich foods, taken from the CSPI fiber scorecard, is presented on page 116.

As you begin to increase consumption of fruits, vegetables, and grains, your intake of dietary fiber will also increase. For example, five to nine daily servings of virtually any fruits and vegetables will contribute quite a few grams of fiber to your diet. Virtually any inclusion of whole-grain bread or beans in the daily diet will easily increase the daily intake of fiber to well within the healthy level of twenty-five to thirty-five grams.

But a final word of caution is in order here. It is especially important to *introduce high-fiber foods into the diet slowly, as we have discussed before regarding other dietary changes.* Many women will find it unacceptable to experience excessive intestinal gas, bloating, or possible diarrhea resulting from too much fiber. Constipation can occasionally occur as well, particularly if inadequate liquids are taken with high-fiber foods or supplements. Nevertheless, the intestinal bacteria responsible for these adverse side effects gradually adjust to the increased fiber load and unpleasant symptoms soon decrease or disappear altogether.

Strategy Number 7: Find *Substitutes* for Fattier Foods

The strategy of substitution has become a guiding principle in any intelligent approach to nutrition and disease prevention. This is because people, health-conscious or not, rarely find it acceptable to eliminate entirely a certain food choice they enjoy. Most of us would prefer to substitute a food item that in some ways resembles the unacceptable food but that has a healthier low-fat profile. For example, consider the following low-fat alternatives offered by Jane E. Brody in a recent *New York Times* article:

LOW-FAT FOOD CHOICE	INSTEAD OF
Pretzels	Chips and nuts
Hot-air popped corn	Microwave or oil-popped corn
Graham crackers or fig bars	Chocolate-chip and nut cookies
Low-fat breads or muffins	Cakes and doughnuts
Crispbreads or flat breads	Regular crackers
Pita or bagel	Croissant
Plain whole-grain cereal	Granola
Fruit spreads or jams	Butter and cream cheese
Mustard or catsup	Mayonnaise
Baked turkey or chicken breast	Bologna and salami
Turkey ham	Hot dogs and sausage
Canadian bacon	Bacon
Extralean ground beef	Regular ground beef

Sirloin-tip roast	T-bone or chuck steak
Nonfat frozen yogurt	Ice cream
Low-fat or skim milk	Whole milk or half-and-half
Low-fat or nonfat yogurt	Sour cream
Low-fat ricotta cheese	Ricotta cheese (whole milk)
Farmer cheese	Cream cheese
Part-skim mozzarella cheese	Muenster or cheddar
Water-packed tuna	Oil-packed fish
Cod, flounder	Salmon or mackerel
Baked or broiled fish	Breaded and fried fish
Tomato sauce	Cream sauce

Many of the choices in the right-hand column can occasionally be eaten if they are prepared according to a low-fat strategy. For example, many cuts of beef can be thoroughly trimmed of excess fat; canned salmon can be made with a nonfat mayonnaise dressing; and several other items can be eaten in limited amounts. Each of these steps will lower the fat content of the entire meal.

Fortunately, the food industry is responding rapidly to some consumers' demands for these kinds of substitutions. According to Christopher Brune, food writer and industry analyst, at least thirty to thirty-five new low-fat, low-cholesterol food products are introduced each month. This rate has not decreased for some years. As Brune tells us, "The health concern is still there, [and] manufacturers are working to improve the flavor of light foods." He adds, "If you really make it taste good, the consumer will buy it."

Many companies such as Smithfield Foods, a manufacturer of processed meats, and Dean Foods Company, manufacturer of dairy products, are joining this attempt to satisfy consumers who want lower-fat food choices. Even Tyson has introduced a line of frozen dinners called Healthy Portion, which just scored high marks in a survey by the Center for Science in the Public Interest.

Pepperidge Farm has introduced a line of six low-fat cookies and two low-fat crackers under the label Healthy Choice, one of which (the low-fat Raspberry Tart) has become one of the company's ten best-selling cookies! Even such a major food producer as Hormel, maker of dozens of meat products bursting with fat, is aware that there is a growing segment of women unwilling to take home these fat-laden items to their families.

The strategy of substitution can be successfully carried out on many fronts. For example:

- *Meats:* Substitute vegetable-based dishes for meat-based ones or simply reduce the amount of meat in the recipes. Always choose lower-fat cuts of meat, such as chicken breast or white-meat turkey. Recognize that turkey burger or sausage is made with a higher percentage of dark meat and skin and therefore has a higher fat content than turkey breast.
- *Dairy:* Avoid whole-milk products whenever possible by choosing 1% fat or skim-milk products. Almost any milk-based product has a low-fat alternative.
- *Snacks:* Avoid fried snacks of any type; instead substitute fruit, air-popped popcorn, pretzels, low-fat crackers, or baked corn chips with a fat-free dip.
- *Sauces:* Several tasty sauces can be easily prepared or purchased in place of the cream-based sauces we normally use.
- *Vegetables:* Substitute lightly steamed or raw vegetables in many of your recipes. They should not be overcooked or sautéed with a lot of oil. As a rule, avoid avocado and coconut.

We conclude this chapter with a brief discussion of healthier approaches you can take to the eating of meat products. While we do not believe that you must become a vegetarian in order to eat a breast-healthy diet, you *will* have to avoid those meats and meat products that are high in fat. As always, you will need to make educated choices and substitutions. The following table compares the fat and calorie content of a variety of commonly eaten meats. In each case, we have listed the contents from 3.5 ounces of the meat. You will notice that there are many choices you can make to improve the nutritional content of a given cut of meat.

This table helps you to understand why eating meat frequently can so easily change your diet from a low-fat to a high-fat pattern.

COMPARING THE FAT CONTENT
OF DIFFERENT CUTS OF MEAT

Type of Meat (3.5 oz.)	High-Fat Method Calories	High-Fat Method Fat Grams	Low-Fat Method Calories	Low-Fat Method Fat Grams
Beef			(excess fat trimmed away)	
Chuck roast	383	30.4	270	15.3
Ground beef, regular	292	20.7		
Rib eye	295	20.6	225	11.6
Top round	211	8.8	191	6.2
Lamb, Pork				
Leg of lamb	276	18.8	184	7.0
Center-loin pork	316	22.1	231	14.9
Lean ham	136	4.9		
Poultry			(without skin)	
Chicken, dark meat	253	15.8	205	9.7
Chicken, light meat	222	10.9	173	4.5
Chicken breast	197	7.9	165	3.0
Turkey, light meat	197	8.3	157	1.2
Duck	337	28.4	201	11.2
Fish				
Flounder	68	0.5		
Mackerel	203	13.8		
Salmon (all types)	210	10.2		
Sea bass	96	2.0		
Shrimp, Lobster	105	1.7		
Tuna, white (in water)	122	1.7		

The table suggests simple ways to reduce both calories and fat grams without having to eliminate meat. Begin to trim away all visible fat, for example, in beef, lamb, or pork. When preparing chicken or turkey, remove the skin whenever possible. And do not forget about serving size: The fat and calorie content can go up quickly if you eat a large serving of any meat.

You will notice, too, that some cuts of beef can be almost as lean as fish and poultry. With a little bit of careful selection and preparation, you will still be able to enjoy some red meat as part of a breast-healthy diet. Do not forget that seafood is also an excellent source of low-fat protein.

All aspects of your diet are open to the process of substitution. Carefully evaluate the lessons you learned during the completion of your food diary. Think about all the meals and snacks you tend to eat and then ask yourself: Do I have to eat the high-fat version or can I make a simple substitution?

RECOMMENDATIONS AND RESOURCES

Throughout this book, we have presented you with the facts and figures that help to explain the links between the foods you choose to eat and your risk for breast cancer. It is vital that every woman put this knowledge to good use—the sooner, the better. Risk reduction should be a priority for *all* women.

We wish we could say with absolute certainty that if you change your diet and your lifestyle, you will never develop a malignant breast tumor. No one can make such a promise. The recommendations in this book are based on observations of breast disease rates in whole populations. At the present time, medical science cannot accurately predict those who will develop breast cancer and those who will not.

Risk reduction does not mean the elimination of every woman's risk for breast cancer. Even in China, Japan, and elsewhere in the world where breast cancer rates are still very low, a small number of women continue to die from this disease. This is what we mean by relative risk: While it can be lowered, it cannot be completely eliminated.

Every woman alive faces this risk, *but not equally*. Our goal is to help you lessen your own individual risk, and you can begin to do so *immediately*. The proper changes in diet and lifestyle could result in tens of thousands of lives saved each year.

Although the entire puzzle of breast cancer prevention is still incomplete, several key pieces are beginning to fit into place. Researchers around the world have performed hundreds of careful studies on the ways diet can reduce the development of malignant breast tumors. Yet it is amazing to find that all too often such valuable information does not filter down to many doctors or their patients.

The challenge in getting this vital message of diet and cancer prevention out to the general public is a difficult one. The problems of communicating health and medical information, even in this era of electronic media, are still enormous. Take, for example, the ongoing effort to substitute lumpectomy as a safe and effective alternative to mastectomy.

In a May 1993 *New York Times* article, entitled "Why Do So Many Women Have Breasts Removed Needlessly?" science writer Gina Kolata maintains that even prominent cancer researchers have difficulty understanding why this important breakthrough has not caught on to a greater extent. "Large highly regarded studies," she writes, "have shown there is rarely any medical reason for amputating a breast rather than simply removing the tumor and treating the breast with a short course of radiation."

Still, mastectomies continue to be performed at high rates. As Dr. I. Craig Henderson, director of breast cancer research at the University of California in San Francisco, explained, "Doctors and patients are not immediately affected by clinical trials." It seems that *a lag of several years* often occurs before a major change in health policy is implemented in response to a series of medical discoveries. Another example is the association between cigarette smoking and lung cancer. This important health message required decades to make the slow transition from medical discovery to a change in public health policy.

Spreading the good news about dietary change and breast cancer risk reduction will no doubt be just as difficult a process. There is public and scientific skepticism to be overcome regarding anything to do with diet or nutrition. There are the endless debates over this or that study and questions concerning study design and the interpretation of results. And there is the political debate surrounding breast cancer research. All of this tends to crowd out the positive message we wish to convey: that *there is indeed strong scientific evidence linking dietary and lifestyle changes to reduced breast cancer risk.*

Women must realize we can't afford the time to sit back and wait another ten or fifteen years for answers. How many more friends and family members will we lose to this illness as we continue to wait? *You* simply cannot risk waiting until the experts are absolutely certain: Breast cancer risk reduction can and ought to begin now.

We recognize the fact that American women have been disappointed time and again by food fads and dietary crazes that claim to make a difference in their health risks. While public wariness is not unjustified, it should not deprive women of hope. A healthy skepticism is justified as long as it does not lead to despair, to the conclusion that there is nothing women can do to reduce their risk.

Those of us in the medical research community who support the National Cancer Institute's Five-a-Day for Better Health program and who advocate the consumption of the specific phytochemical-rich vegetables and fruits outlined here to reduce breast cancer risk will undoubtedly be criticized by those who favor a much more cautious approach to preventive medicine. However, the accumulated scientific evidence is beginning to speak for itself. Hopefully, more and more health professionals will come to see that these guidelines can indeed make a difference in a woman's risk and survival.

Let us, then, summarize the steps you can begin to take *today* to lessen your risk of breast cancer.

The Importance of Early Detection

Breast Exams

The importance to a woman of detecting a malignant breast lump *early* in the course of the illness cannot be overemphasized. And even though we have stressed primary prevention of breast cancer throughout this book, the *first step* each woman must take in reducing her risk is to become fully informed about the importance of *early detection*.

Unfortunately, many women are still too frightened to examine their own breasts, too afraid of what they may find. If you have been hesitant in the past, a good time to start breast self-exams is right after you have received a clean bill of health from your doctor. You will be less fearful of finding something and can then begin to learn how your breasts normally feel. This may help give you the confidence you need to find a possible tumor while it is still small.

You should examine your own breasts at least once a month, approximately five to seven days after your period begins. If you are postmenopausal, find a convenient way to remind yourself to do so every month (for example, the day you receive your phone bill). You should also have a breast examination during your routine medical or gynecological checkups.

The technique of breast self-examination requires a little practice to be most effective, but it is not difficult. The best place to do this is in the shower or bath, where the soapy water increases the sensitivity of your fingers on the skin. Several teaching materials, posters, soft-breast models containing small lumps, and videotapes are available to help you learn this skill. A call to your local branch of the American Cancer Society (national office: 800–ACS–2345) will help you obtain these self-examination aids. Visit your local library to learn of women's health groups in your community.

Routine annual or semiannual gynecological visits should include a thorough breast exam. As a woman gets older (past the age of forty), particularly if she is at higher risk, it is especially important that she have her breasts examined by a health professional on a *routine basis*. These exams should be scheduled even if there aren't any symptoms or other medical complaints at the time.

Mammography

Several recent medical studies have raised the question of the true health benefits of regular mammography before the age of fifty. Since this controversy is not likely to be settled soon, most of the larger organizations continue to adhere to the guidelines proposed over the years by the American Cancer Society and the National Cancer Institute. These can be summarized as follows:

- Most women below the age of thirty-five are not likely to benefit from a mammogram. This is because breast cancer is very infrequent in this age group. In addition, breast tissue is denser at younger ages, making it difficult to pick up early lumps.
- Between the ages of thirty-five and forty, most experts agree that it is a good idea to have a baseline mammogram. This will not only help detect any early abnormalities but will also serve as a useful comparison in later years.
- Between the ages of forty and fifty, a mammogram should be performed every one to two years for most women. If a woman comes from a high-risk family or if she has a large number of the known risk factors, a mammogram is recommended *at least* once a year.
- After the age of fifty, all women will benefit from annual mammograms.

The newer, state-of-the-art mammography machines have reduced the amount of radiation to which you are exposed during these X rays. For this reason, it is valuable to have your mammography performed at a location where the best equipment is available.

The amount of radiation received by the breasts in a regular mammogram is actually quite small, so women should not worry about any danger from the mammogram itself.

An excellent way to locate a qualified and accredited mammography facility near you is to call the American College of Radiology (800–ACR–LINE) or the National Cancer Institute (800–4–CANCER). Another important step is to be certain that the radiologist reading your mammogram is board-certified or board-eligible and that he or she has considerable experience in frequently interpreting these kinds of X rays.

Diet and Lifestyle: The Importance of Exercise

Nearly all of the important benefits obtained by eating phytochemical-rich foods will be further enhanced by exercise. Research studies have shown that women who exercised earlier in their lives are better protected against breast cancer. Physical fitness, after all, is simply the result of performing moderately vigorous exercise *on a regular basis*, without becoming exhausted. Once you have attained a given level of fitness, it is necessary that you maintain it and, if possible, improve upon it throughout your life.

Just as with diet, you will need to begin any exercise program slowly and comfortably. All you need to do at the beginning is to *get moving*. The level of exercise suitable for you will depend on your past exercise experience. For those women who have never been physically active as adults, a good way to start is to begin a walking program.

To ensure the success of any exercise program, however, pay attention to the basics. First, use the right equipment. If walking or aerobic exercise is what you choose to do, then be sure to wear comfortable and durable shoes. Second, make the time. Once begun, your exercise program should not be set aside because you have "more important things" to do. Exercise should be performed *routinely*—at least three times per week for periods of at least twenty to thirty minutes. Other members of your family or household should be aware that this is your personal exercise time. Make sure it is not easily interrupted.

A third basic rule of thumb is always to stretch and warm up properly before beginning any exercise routine. Nothing will set you back further, both practically and emotionally, than an unnecessary turned ankle, pulled muscle, pinched nerve, or swollen joint. Any one of these may occur if you do not first take the time to prepare your muscles fully.

An exercise program does not need to be elaborate in order to meet the goals of providing you with aerobic fitness, flexibility, and strength. All that you truly require is the time and the will to stick with a program you have designed or chosen to meet your own needs.

A Seven-Day Food Plan

On the following few pages, we will suggest a typical week's food plan that can be adopted fairly easily. This food plan draws upon many of the recipes we offer in Chapter 13. Our suggested food plan is rich in phytochemicals and it incorporates all of the dietary strategies discussed in the previous chapter. We offer this plan as an example of just how easy it is to adopt and follow a breast-healthy diet. All items in boldface type can be found in the recipe section beginning on page 181.

Day 1: Monday

Breakfast

> 6-ounce glass of grapefruit juice
> **Stuffed Baked Apple**
> Toasted whole-wheat English muffin with low-fat cottage cheese
>   or part-skim ricotta cheese
> 6-ounce glass of 1% or skim milk

Lunch

Salmon Salad
Hard roll with shredded lettuce
Plum tomatoes and cucumber slices
Pear or fresh peach
Lemonade, tea, coffee, or fruit juice

Dinner

Hearty Cabbage Soup
French bread—2 slices
Sweet-and-Sour Veggies
Brown rice
Rainbow sherbet with blueberries
Beverage

Nutritional assessment:

Total calories	1,609
Grams of fat	20
Grams of fiber	29
Vitamin A (RE)	2,590
Vitamin C (mg)	208
Calcium (mg)	790
% fat calories	11%
Fruit/vegetable servings	7

Other tips: Stuffed baked apples can be made in advance and kept in the refrigerator until eaten. When possible, use high-fiber breads and rolls in all your meals.

Day 2: Tuesday

Breakfast

6-ounce glass of orange juice
Toasted bagel with farmer cheese or nonfat cream cheese mixed
   with finely chopped green pepper, red pepper, radishes
½ cup of applesauce
1% milk (6 ounces)
Coffee, tea

Lunch

6-ounce glass of tomato juice with slice of lemon
Greek salad: chopped tomatoes, cucumber, radishes, green pep-
   per, lettuce, Greek black olives (four, diced), cubed feta
   cheese, low-fat or nonfat dressing
Toasted whole-wheat pita bread (6 inches)
Iced tea or coffee

Dinner

½ grapefruit, center filled with grapes
Turkey Cutlets with Spicy Fruit Sauce
Red potatoes boiled (microwaved) in skins, served with nonfat
   sour cream or yogurt and chopped fresh dill
Steamed broccoli (about 1 cup)
2 slices whole-wheat bread
Ice milk with sliced strawberries

Nutritional assessment:

Total calories	1,651
Grams of fat	21
Grams of fiber	28
Vitamin A (RE)	965
Vitamin C (mg)	401

Calcium (mg)	855
% fat calories	11%
Fruit/vegetable servings	11

Other tips: Try using green tea as a beverage, in place of coffee or ordinary tea. It is great hot or cold.

Day 3: Wednesday

Breakfast

6-ounce glass of tomato juice
Bowl of whole-wheat cereal (about 6 ounces—add ¼ cup of raisins and ⅛ cup of dry-roasted soy nuts)
6 ounces 1% milk
Tea or coffee

Lunch

V-8 juice (6 ounces)
White-meat turkey breast on rye bread, Dijon mustard, sliced tomato and lettuce, low-fat or nonfat dressing
Apple
Iced tea, coffee, or mineral water

Dinner

Orange slices
Oriental Chicken Platter
Brown rice
Chinese Cole Slaw
Fresh pineapple chunks (or, if unavailable, canned in their own juice)
Coffee or tea

Nutritional assessment:

Total calories	1,424
Grams of fat	29
Grams of fiber	30
Vitamin A (RE)	1,225
Vitamin C (mg)	280
Calcium (mg)	705
% fat calories	18%
Fruit/vegetable servings	8

Other tips: An alternative dessert is an ice-milk shake. Blend any fresh or frozen fruit with low-fat or nonfat ice cream or yogurt. Just remember that low in fat does not always mean low in calories.

Day 4: Thursday

Breakfast

6-ounce glass of orange juice
Two slices of rye toast with nonfat cream cheese and all-fruit jam
1 banana, sliced, with low-fat sour cream or yogurt
Coffee, tea, 1% milk (6 ounces)

Lunch

Fresh fruit salad with low-fat (or nonfat) yogurt or cottage cheese
Toasted pita or hard roll (whole-wheat)
Seltzer water with lemon or 100% fruit juice
Two low-fat cookies (for example, Pepperidge Farm Healthy Choice, or Snack-Well)

Dinner

Karen's Vegetable Soup
Tofu Lasagna
Carrots in Consommé
Grissini (low-fat, thin Italian bread sticks)
Slice of cantaloupe with raspberry sorbet
Beverage

Nutritional assessment:

Total calories	1,624
Grams of fat	16
Grams of fiber	24
Vitamin A (RE)	5,175
Vitamin C (mg)	222
Calcium (mg)	1,389
% fat calories	9%
Fruit/vegetable servings	8–9

Day 5: Friday

Breakfast

6-ounce glass of 100% apple juice
¾ cup of whole-grain cereal with ½ cup of fresh fruit (e.g.,
    berries, peaches, grapes, cantaloupe chunks)
6 ounces 1% milk
Coffee or tea

Lunch

Cup of **Karen's Vegetable Soup** (left over from Thursday)
Thin-sliced roast beef sandwich on rye or whole-wheat bread
    with shredded lettuce and tomato and Dijon mustard
Tangerine

Iced tea, coffee, fruit juice
Low-fat yogurt (6 ounces) with sprinkling of wheat bran or raisins

Dinner

Cabbage Fruit Delight
Chicken with Broccoli
Brown rice
French or Italian bread
Apple with a slice of low-fat cheese
Tea

Nutritional assessment:
Total calories	1,611
Grams of fat	26
Grams of fiber	31
Vitamin A (RE)	2,185
Vitamin C (mg)	251
Calcium (mg)	1,048
% fat calories	15%
Fruit/vegetable servings	7

Day 6: Saturday

Breakfast

6-ounce glass of apricot nectar
Skinny French Toast
½ cup of fresh fruit (cut up)
Coffee, tea, or 1% milk with fat-free chocolate syrup

Lunch

Cup of low-salt, nonfat canned lentil and carrot soup (e.g.,
Pritikin or Healthy Valley)

Large tomato stuffed with tuna salad, low-fat dressing, set on a
   bed of mixed salad greens
Cabbage Fruit Delight (left over from Friday)
Peach
Iced coffee or iced tea with lemon

Dinner

Salad of arugula, endive, chicory, tomatoes, and olives in a spicy
   low-fat or nonfat dressing
Italian-Style Chicken Cutlets
Linguini Primavera
Italian bread
Fruit ices
Cappuccino, regular coffee, or tea

Nutritional assessment:

Total calories	1,624
Grams of fat	35
Grams of fiber	30
Vitamin A (RE)	2,340
Vitamin C (mg)	314
Calcium (mg)	634
% fat calories	19%
Fruit/vegetable servings	8

Other tips: In your salads, select whatever mixed greens are
available. Try substituting small amounts of red-leaf lettuce, dandelion greens, or kale.

Day 7: Sunday

Breakfast

6-ounce glass of orange juice
2 slices of whole-wheat bread with all-fruit jam

Vegetable Omelet
Wedge of cantaloupe, honeydew melon, or watermelon
Coffee, tea, or 1% (or skim) milk

Lunch

Low-fat ham and cheese sandwich on rye bread with Dijon mustard
Carrot sticks and pickle slices (or olives)
Cranberry juice with club soda
Bunch of grapes

Dinner

Tossed green salad and assorted fresh vegetables with tangy low-fat or nonfat salad dressing
Spaghetti with Meat Sauce
Cauliflower Italiano
Italian bread
Beverage
2 small fresh plums

Nutritional assessment:

Total calories	1,653
Grams of fat	36
Grams of fiber	24
Vitamin A (RE)	3,291
Vitamin C (mg)	367
Calcium (mg)	744
% fat calories	20%
Fruit/vegetable servings	7–8

Recipes and Cookbooks

At some point, you will undoubtedly want to try other new recipes
and will look for a good cookbook. Be prepared: A visit to your local

bookstore or library to find a cookbook can be an overwhelming experience. You will encounter an amazing number and variety of books. Because of the enormous number of attractive choices, you may be unable to decide which cookbook is most suitable for you.

In our opinion, you would do well to choose from those cookbooks that try to educate you about food contents and food values. It is crucial that you learn to recognize and prepare breast-healthy recipes. Your task will be easier if you choose a cookbook designed with your health in mind.

Here is a sampling of some excellent cookbooks that provide nutritional information along with their recipes.

Cooking Light Cookbook 1993
Oxmoor House, Inc., 1992
Book Division of Southern Progress Corp.
Birmingham, AL

The Eating Well Cookbook
Edited by Rux Martin, Patricia Johnson, and Elizabeth Hiser
Camden House Publishing, Inc., 1991
Charlotte, VT

These two enjoyable cookbooks, along with their namesake magazines, contain much more than just recipes.

Prevention's Super Foods Cookbook—250 Delicious Recipes Using Nature's Healthiest Foods
Rodale Press, Inc., 1993
Emmaus, PA

This cookbook was compiled by the food editors of *Prevention* magazine.

Weight Watchers Favorite Homestyle Recipes
Penguin Books, 1993

These recipes have been compiled by the nutritional staff of Weight Watchers International, Inc., who have been focusing on healthy eating for years.

Graham Kerr's Minimax Cookbook
Doubleday, 1992

Low Fat & Loving It
Ruth Spear
Warner Books, 1991

Great Good Food, Luscious Lower-Fat Cooking
Julee Rosso
Crown, 1993

All three of these cookbooks are excellent sources of healthy, enjoyable recipes, with lots of cooking tips.

The New Vegetarian Cookbook
Gary Null
MacMillan, 1980

The Classic Vegetable Cookbook
Ruth Spear
Harper & Row, 1985

The Tofu Book
John Paino and Lisa Messinger
Nasoya Foods, Inc.
23 Jytek Drive, Leominster, MA 01453
(508–537–0713)

These last three books are not as well documented as the others when it comes to nutritional information. However, with vegetarian cooking, it's hard to go wrong. We include them because they are a good source of vegetable dishes, particularly more soybean-tofu recipes.

Helpful Guides and Tools

There are several fact-filled aids that you can put to good use right away. Many of these are available from the Center for Science in the Public Interest (CSPI). First is CSPI's *Nutrition Action Health Letter*. It can be obtained by writing the central office at 1875 Connecticut Avenue, N.W., Suite 300, Washington, D.C. 20009–5728 or by calling 202–332–9110.

CSPI also offers a variety of tools to help analyze your foods at a glance. These include slide charts for the fat and fiber content of over 240 common foods, laminated posters, computer software for analyzing the nutritional content of thousands of commonly available foods, and several videotapes. All of these can be obtained by writing CSPI or calling the aforementioned number.

Two other valuable health newsletters are the *Tufts University Diet & Nutrition Letter* (P.O. Box 57834, Boulder, CO 80321–7834), and the *University of California, Berkeley Wellness Letter* (P.O. Box 420148, Palm Coast, FL 32142).

In addition to cookbooks, many women have found fat- and calorie-counting books helpful for comparisons. Some of the more complete guides are listed below.

The Complete Book of Food Counts
Corinne T. Netzer
Dell Publishing, 1991
$5.99, paperback

Dr. Bruce Lowell's Fat % Finder
Bruce K. Lowell
Perigee Books, 1991
$8.95, paperback

The Corinne T. Netzer Fat Gram Counter
Corinne T. Netzer
Dell Publishing, 1992
$4.99, paperback

The Quick and Easy Fat Gram and Calorie Counter
Lynn Sonberg
Avon Books, 1992
$3.99, paperback

——————————

Chapter Twelve

QUESTIONS AND ANSWERS

We offer the following chapter as the most direct way to address the questions you may have after reading our book. Our answers are based on the most up-to-date medical information available.

Several women in my family have had breast cancer. Will I get it, too?

The probability of developing breast cancer is never 100 percent. Even if many members of your family have already had this disease, you still may not have inherited the faulty gene. Moreover, a single genetic defect, inherited through your family, probably isn't sufficient by itself to cause a malignancy. Other DNA damage during your life must also occur, and you may be able to prevent some of it.

It is important to understand that you should not be frightened into inaction by your family's experience with breast cancer. A woman's risk can always be lowered to some degree. The best way to begin reducing that risk is through breast-healthy changes in diet and lifestyle.

If there is a man in my family who had breast cancer, or a woman on my father's side with the disease, does that raise my risk?

Male family members who have developed breast cancer contribute to your genetic risk in the same way as the female family members do. Also, if women on your father's side of the family have breast cancer, it is certainly possible that a genetic trait, hidden in your father, has been passed along to you. Breast cancer specialists usually place more emphasis on your mother's family, since the possible presence of a familial breast cancer trait will be more evident among the women.

I've already had breast cancer once. Can I get it again?

Breast cancer is not like an infectious disease, where lifelong immunity follows from an early bout of the disease. A woman is still at risk for this disease throughout the remainder of her life. A previous breast tumor *increases* a woman's risk for developing a second tumor. This is presumably because whatever originally prompted her breast cells to become malignant probably also adversely affected many more of her breast cells.

Nevertheless, we must repeat again: *All women* can reduce their risk for breast cancer, regardless of where they are starting from. Careful dietary choices will undoubtedly help you, even if you were previously treated for a breast malignancy.

I was told that my breast cancer was estrogen-negative. Can a careful diet protect me, anyway?

When used in connection with breast cancer, the term *estrogen-negative* indicates that a tumor is not as sensitive to the presence of estrogen as *estrogen-positive* tumors. The estrogen-negative breast tumors have low levels of the estrogen receptor; consequently, such drugs as tamoxifen have much less effect on them. However, even estrogen-negative breast tumors will benefit from a phytochemical-rich diet.

If you recall, we pointed out in Chapter 8 that carotenoids are capable of protecting the breast and that they work by mechanisms other than the modification of estrogen. There can be literally thousands of different phytochemicals in a diet high in fruits, grains, and vegetables. Many of these plant substances act by elevating the presence of protective enzymes, by functioning as antioxidants, by encouraging noncancerous growth of cells, and by inactivating potential toxic substances in the breasts. Each of these processes could potentially benefit your estrogen-negative tumor.

Tumor processes in various other organs of the body are similarly slowed down by the phytochemicals in a healthy diet. It is clear that five to nine servings of fruits and vegetables per day, practiced consistently throughout one's life, will slow the growth not only of hormone-positive and hormone-negative breast cancers but also the growth of malignant cells throughout the body.

How does smoking affect my risk for breast cancer?

While smoking was found to reduce the risk of estrogen-dependent endometrial cancer, it did not similarly lower the risk of breast cancer. Any positive hormonal value of cigarettes is offset by the toxic properties of the cigarette smoke itself. Women should realize that tobacco smoke contains over five hundred potentially toxic substances created in the burning ember of the cigarette. Many of these hazardous substances are eventually secreted into the breast ducts, where they can affect the breast cells lining the ducts. Some of these toxins will be transferred by the milk to a breast-feeding infant.

Therefore, while most studies indicate smoking neither lowers nor raises a woman's risk for breast cancer, the overall effect of smoking on the breast is a negative one. The presence of these toxins near the breast cells can only be viewed as a danger.

Do breast implants increase my risk for developing a malignant breast tumor?

The question of health risks from silicone breast implants has grown considerably in recent years, spurred on by widespread media coverage and the ever-increasing numbers of women undergoing this medical procedure.

Fortunately, there is little to no evidence at this time that *intact* silicone implants cause an additional risk for breast cancer. There is some concern, however, that implants may interfere both with breast examination and mammography.

The most serious problem for women with implants comes from a possible rupture of the fluid-filled device. Silicone is itself inert and nontoxic. Yet once an implant has ruptured, the presence of silicone seeping around the breast tissue may cause local inflammation and irritation to the breast ducts. Some scientists believe that any chronic inflammation to a tissue may be a setup for a later tumor. In order to remain safe, any woman with a breast implant must be sure to be examined frequently by her physician.

Does breast size have anything to do with breast cancer?

Researchers have found that large breast size does not necessarily mean that a woman is more likely to form a breast tumor. However, there are some circumstances where large breasts may be detrimental to a woman's efforts to prevent breast cancer.

For example, very large breasts may interfere with both mammography and breast examination. It is possible that a smaller tumor, usually picked up in most women, will be missed in a large-breasted woman, to be found only at a later date, when it has had a greater chance of spreading. Also, large breasts are associated with obesity in some women, and this *is* a risk factor for breast cancer.

Is a high cholesterol level linked to breast cancer?

High cholesterol levels are not known to be *directly* linked to breast cancer. On the other hand, dietary habits known to increase serum cholesterol (for example, increased amounts of animal fat) are probably harmful to the breasts, as well.

Heart disease, breast cancer, and colon cancer are all considered diseases of the West. Each of these diseases seems to have a strong dietary component, linked to high fat (and low vegetable/fruit) intake common in Western nations. These illnesses are believed to be helped by a dietary regime that is low in fat and high in fruit and vegetable fiber. Most dietary recommendations aimed at lowering cholesterol will generally be consistent with those suggested for reducing breast cancer risk.

Should a woman become pregnant if she has already been treated for breast cancer?

This is a difficult question to answer, since a young woman who has had breast cancer can feel torn between the desire to have a child and the need to protect herself. During pregnancy, enormous amounts of estrogen are produced; these hormones greatly stimulate the breast. The breast normally grows rapidly during pregnancy in preparation for the upcoming birth. As you learned in Chapter 2, having a full-term pregnancy can indeed protect the breasts. It does so by encouraging the breasts to fully mature, or "differentiate." If, however, the hormonal stimulation of pregnancy occurs after tumor cells are present, a woman's risks are different.

In a young woman with a personal history of breast cancer, the risk is that any malignant cells still in her body are going to be overly stimulated by these high hormone levels. This is a complex dilemma with no easy solution. Any woman making the choice to bear a child under these circumstances should be closely supervised by her physician throughout her pregnancy.

Does electromagnetic radiation from electric power lines cause an additional risk for breast cancer?

As part of the ongoing search for modifiable causes of breast cancer, many have questioned the potential risks of high-power electrical wires near their homes. This is a source of continuing controversy. Much of the early research was concerned with the possible link of electric wires and childhood leukemia. In general, medical researchers find the evidence linking this form of radiation to breast cancer to be incomplete and inconclusive. Further research in this area will need to be carefully designed and controlled if it is to arrive at a conclusion convincing to those on both sides of this debate.

Is drinking lots of coffee harmful to my breasts?

Most breast cancer scientists see little cancer danger to the breasts from coffee and other caffeine-containing beverages. Nevertheless, coffee has a long-standing reputation for exacerbating pain from fibrocystic breasts.

Coffee is used so widely by so many millions of women that its overall safety can hardly be questioned. Several careful scientific studies of this question have been performed, but the results have been inconclusive. This fact alone tells us that any risk from caffeine is probably too small to detect.

Yet many women still feel strongly that limiting coffee intake alleviates their symptoms of breast tenderness and swelling each month. Moderate use of coffee or similar beverages probably poses little risk to most women.

How dangerous to the breasts is the radiation I get from a mammogram?

As the importance of screening mammograms has grown, radiologists and other scientists have worked hard at making mammography machines more efficient at much lower doses of radiation. Their continuing efforts have had the real benefit of making mammograms safer than ever. To understand the issue of mammogram safety, you must compare the *possible risk* with the *actual benefit* of a mammogram.

There is certainly some risk involved anytime you get an X ray, even though that risk may be very small. In the case of mammography, it has been estimated that about one in every 25,000 women undergoing the procedure will get just enough radiation to push her breast cells over the limit, thereby starting a breast tumor. But compare this with the fact that all of those 25,000 women will benefit from knowing whether or not an early malignancy exists that requires prompt attention. Obviously, the benefits to your health far outweigh the small risk involved. And year by year, with advanced technology, the already small risk of mammography will become even smaller still.

How is my risk affected if I took estrogen for only a short period in my life?

The danger from any potential cancer-causing substance in the body depends mostly on the *amount* and the *duration* of your exposure. For example, we all know breathing the diesel exhaust fumes coming from a city bus is not good for us. Fortunately, however, we are near the bus for only a few moments; the net danger, therefore, is likely to be insignificant. It is a long-standing cumulative exposure that matters most.

Similarly, the risk to your breasts from a relatively short-term exposure to additional estrogen (either oral contraceptives or post-menopausal estrogen therapy) is minimal. Most scientific studies of this topic have found that additional cancer risk to your breasts only becomes evident after approximately five years of use.

The overall added danger from oral contraceptives or hormone replacement therapy is not as great as that of some other risk factors (see the table on page 30). Nevertheless, many millions of women are taking these medications at any given time. The best advice at present is to limit your *long-term use* of additional hormones when possible. If necessary, you should consult your physician or gynecologist about alternatives.

Is there danger to the breasts from the hormones used during in vitro fertilization, particularly since the procedure is often done more than once?

The use of fertility drugs is usually not associated with an increased risk for breast cancer. Most of these agents are taken on just a few occasions rather than chronically over a sustained period of time. In some cases, a woman may experience some hormonal changes in her body, including her breasts. However, this is only temporary and it will subside.

My doctor insists I need estrogen therapy. Is it still possible to lower my risk even though I take estrogen?

Yes, it is possible to continue to lower your risk for breast cancer if you are taking some form of hormonal supplementation. We have already discussed some of the risks associated with additional estrogen. The protective effects of phytochemicals in your diet will continue to benefit you even under these circumstances. It is important to realize, however, that the dosage of supplemental estrogen may need to be adjusted if you make rapid changes in your diet. The reason is that many of the phytochemicals in a diet high in fruits and vegetables can stimulate the metabolic enzymes in the liver and intestines. Under some circumstances, this fact may slightly alter the effectiveness of some drugs, including estrogen.

Are mammograms fail-safe? How can I be sure that I am getting a good mammogram and that the doctor has not missed something?

Some areas of the breast cannot be well visualized on mammograms. Tumors forming in those areas (near the borders of the breast and up toward the armpits) may be missed. Furthermore, some tumors that can be felt by a woman or her doctor will occasionally not show up on breast X rays. This may happen more often in young women, since any suspicious lump is likely to be small and the surrounding breast tissue frequently dense, thus hiding any small tumors.

You must take the proper steps to know that your mammogram is being done by skilled personnel using the best available machines. The phone numbers listed in the previous chapter will help you find a center accredited by the American College of Radiology. It is also a good rule of thumb to consult a radiologist who spends much of the time looking at mammograms.

If I am getting my mammograms regularly, do I really have to continue to examine my own breasts?

A common misconception is that since mammograms are so much more efficient at finding smaller tumors, routine breast exams have become rather pointless. This is far from true.

First of all, mammograms are performed in many women only on a yearly basis, and often much less frequently than that. During all the intervening months since her last mammogram, a woman has an ongoing opportunity to examine herself for the possibility of an unusual lump.

There are other reasons to continue being examined. For one thing, regular breast exams by a health professional help assure you that you are doing it correctly. Also, mammograms do not evaluate all of the breast tissue, as we have seen. Those regions of the breasts near the chest wall are not easily fitted under the machine. It is, therefore, still important that you be examined.

We realize breast exams are frightening to many women and that it sometimes takes only a small excuse to avoid this preventive measure. Each woman needs to face up to her own reluctance as best she can. We hope to convince you that there is much you can do to keep a malignant breast tumor from ever forming. By knowing about and acting on such positive news, perhaps more women will be encouraged to practice self-examination as part of a comprehensive approach to a breast-healthy diet and lifestyle.

If estrogen is so involved with breast cancer, should I have my levels checked?

A single blood test to determine estrogen levels gives your physician little information about your ongoing hormonal stimulation. This is because estrogen normally fluctuates between fairly low and high levels in the bloodstream throughout the menstrual cycle. During some cycles, the fluctuations will be greater than in other months. A single test, therefore, taken without regard to the day of the menstrual cycle, will be difficult to interpret.

In older women, monthly hormonal fluctuations are no longer a problem. Since estrogen levels in older women fall to very low levels, many labs are not able to make these specialized measurements. For all these reasons, physicians generally do not measure estrogen levels in most woman unless there is a specific hormonal problem to evaluate. Such measurements may be beneficial as a part of a comprehensive evaluation and plan geared toward reducing your risk. But as a single test, measurement of your estrogen levels has little screening value.

Is there any chance that my estrogen levels can fall too low if I eat a diet high in fruits, grains, and vegetables?

Given the powerful nature of many of the phytochemicals present in the foods we can eat, it would not be surprising if a woman's hormone levels occasionally fell too low. However, this is rarely the case.

Some research studies have observed that switching to a completely vegetarian diet occasionally alters a woman's menstrual cycle, speeding it up or delaying it by a few days. In research studies, the shift to a different dietary pattern is relatively sudden. In the real world, your dietary changes are made much more gradually. When dietary habits are altered slowly, your body has the opportunity to adjust to them over time.

Some women eating a breast-healthy diet will experience a small decrease in their menstrual flow due to the fact that the uterus is not being encouraged to proliferate as extensively. This is not known to be associated with decreased fertility.

Indeed, a breast-healthy diet rarely causes the body's hormone levels to fall too low. This is probably because the different phytochemicals each act in slightly different ways, no one of them overwhelming any aspect of the Estrogen Pathway. Also, many of the phytochemicals act by transforming estrogen into a safer form (for example, C-2 and not C-16) rather than eliminating it altogether from the body.

I am beginning to eat more fruits and vegetables, but I feel bloated from gas. Will this ever diminish?

One of the biggest obstacles to eating more fruits, grains, beans, and vegetables is the fear of uncomfortable intestinal side effects. Women who have never attempted to eat the required five to nine servings of these foods each day may experience the most discomfort.

However, it's important to understand that our bodies have evolved over thousands of years along with these plant foods, and that our digestive systems are quite capable of digesting far more phytochemical-rich foods than we normally eat. You can be confident your body will fully adjust to this new eating pattern relatively soon (as little as two to three weeks). After that point, you will find there will be far more trouble with indigestion should you return to your old high-fat foods.

In the meantime, be patient with your body. It took you many years to develop the pattern of eating fatty foods. Give yourself the time needed to adjust to a breast-healthy pattern.

How do phytochemicals hold up to microwaving and other types of cooking?

One of the most commonly asked questions concerns the effects of cooking on plant chemicals and vitamins. Some phytochemicals actually increase in concentration when the vegetable is cooked: The best examples are vitamin A and other carotenoids. However, many phytochemicals will be lost when overcooked.

Various cooking methods have different effects on the phytochemicals present in a vegetable or fruit. Garlic, for example, can be minced, sautéed, boiled, or added in dry form. Each method will yield a slightly different phytochemical profile.

It is impossible at this point in our knowledge to be certain about the best cooking technique for every vegetable. Follow this simple rule: Whenever possible, *keep it crisp.* If you microwave or steam a vegetable, try not to overdo it. Extended boiling of vegetables is probably the most damaging to their phytochemical contents. The key is not to overcook them. Steaming vegetables is the preferred alternative.

I eat a fairly healthy diet, yet my breasts still get tender and swollen each month. Am I doing something wrong?

Some women are much more prone to these symptoms than others, a condition sometimes referred to as fibrocystic disease. If you recall, this really isn't a disease at all. However, the presence of this condition does suggest that your breasts may be getting overstimulated each month.

All of the strategies outlined throughout this book will act over time to decrease the proliferation and tenderness of your breasts. It may simply take more time and effort for one woman than it would for another. For women plagued with this recurrent condition, we offer the following recommendations.

First of all, be sure you are up to date with your regular screening routine, including breast exams and mammography. Second, attempt to lower your dietary fat to well below 20 percent of calories and to increase your consumption of the kinds of vegetables discussed in Chapter 8.

The third-most-important step you can take *right now* is to create your own exercise program. The combination of a diet very low in fat and high in phytochemicals and an active *aerobic* program will certainly decrease the ongoing stimulation to your breast cells.

Chapter Thirteen

RECIPES

Most of the recipes in this chapter have been included because of the abundant supply of breast-healthy phytochemicals they offer. These recipes offer you various ways to incorporate indole-rich crucifers, isoflavone-rich soybeans, and carotenoid-rich vegetables into the meals you prepare and eat each day. We have included both entrée items as well as side dishes.

Recognize that most of these recipes can be modified by varying the vegetables and dressings. For example, when the recipe calls for green bell peppers, feel free to substitute the red or yellow varieties. Or try different types of cabbage and different types of salad greens.

You will also notice that some recipes call for tofu. We recommend that you spend some time going to several of your local health-food stores to determine which has the best variety of tofu. Most large supermarket chains usually carry at least one brand. Find the extrafirm and lower-fat varieties, if possible.

Along with each recipe is a selected summary of its basic nutritional contents. Recipes were analyzed using Dine Right software, developed by DINE Systems, Inc., 586 North French Road, Suite 2, Amherst, New York 14228 (716–688–2492). The software can also be purchased from the Center for Science in the Public Interest (CSPI), 1875 Connecticut Avenue, N.W., Suite 300, Washington, D.C. 20009–5728.

Bon Appétit!

Baked Honey Squash

1 squash (acorn or butternut is best)
cinnamon and nutmeg
2 tablespoons brown sugar or honey

Carefully slice the squash into two halves lengthwise. Scoop out the seeds and tough fiber and discard. Sprinkle cinnamon, nutmeg, and a tablespoon of brown sugar or honey on each of the squash halves. Cover each half with a small piece of aluminum foil.

Put the squash halves in a preheated 350°F oven for about 1 hour. To test if done, lift the foil and pierce the flesh with a fork. If it is soft, it's ready to eat.

Each half squash serves one. Nutritional information per serving: 169 calories, 1 gram of fat, 6 grams of dietary fiber, 89 RE of vitamin A, 23 milligrams vitamin C.

Variations: Try adding a few chopped nuts (for example, walnuts) and ¼ cup of raisins to each half of squash about 15 minutes before serving.

Strawberry Spinach Salad

⅓ cup reduced-calorie or nonfat salad dressing
¼ cup orange juice
1 teaspoon sugar
1 teaspoon poppy seeds
½ pound fresh spinach, washed carefully, trimmed, and torn into
    pieces
2 cups fresh sliced strawberries (remove the hulls)

Combine the first four ingredients in a small bowl; stir well and set aside. Gently toss the spinach and strawberries in a large bowl. Drizzle the poppy seed mixture over them.

Serves three. Nutritional information per serving: 97 calories, 1 gram of fat, 6 grams of dietary fiber, 515 RE of vitamin A, 89 milligrams vitamin C.

Cauliflower Italiano

1 small head cauliflower (cleaned, about 4 cups)
vegetable-oil spray
1 cup seasoned bread crumbs
salt and pepper to taste
1 tablespoon margarine (⅛ of a stick)
6 ounces part-skim-milk mozzarella cheese, grated

Separate cauliflower into flowerets, discarding much of the inner stem and leaves. Steam for 3 to 4 minutes. Do not overcook, because you want the cauliflower to maintain a firm texture. When finished, remove from heat and set aside. Using the vegetable-oil spray, grease a casserole dish thoroughly. Dust the casserole with half of the bread crumbs.

Add the cauliflower, season lightly with salt and pepper, and sprinkle in the remaining bread crumbs. Dot with small pieces of the margarine and the grated mozzarella cheese.

This dish can be made in advance and refrigerated. Bake, uncovered, for 25 minutes at 350°F. If desired, decorate when serving with a few sliced black olives.

Serves four. Nutritional information per serving: 227 calories, 8 grams of fat, 3 grams of dietary fiber, 88 RE of vitamin A, 68 milligrams vitamin C.

Variations: Try garnishing with 2 tablespoons of chopped red pimento right before serving. Another popular garnish is a few sprigs of fresh parsley or cilantro on the side. However, don't forget that these are not on the dish merely to look at: They can be eaten, as well.

Confetti Coleslaw

4 cups shredded cabbage (red and green)
½ cup chopped green pepper
½ cup chopped red sweet pepper
½ cup grated carrots
¼ cup finely chopped onion
½ cup shredded red radishes

Dressing:
¼–½ cup apple juice or cider
2 tablespoons fresh dill chopped or two teaspoons bottled dill weed
2 teaspoons prepared mustard (e.g., Dijon)
6 tablespoons light (low-fat) mayonnaise or salad dressing
salt and pepper to taste

Combine the ingredients for the dressing and toss with the cabbage and the other vegetables to blend. If possible, refrigerate for a couple of hours before serving.

Serves six. Nutritional information per serving: 78 calories, 0–4 grams of fat (depending on dressing), 2 grams of dietary fiber, 313 RE of vitamin A, 55 milligrams vitamin C.

Variations: In this dish, you can mix up the types of cabbage for different flavors. The standard green or the crinkly green type, known as savoy, can both be used. Use different amounts of red cabbage for variety and color. Note that all fat can be eliminated from this recipe with the use of a nonfat salad dressing.

Cabbage Fruit Delight

1 small green cabbage, thinly shredded (about 4 cups)
½ cup seedless grapes (cut in halves)
1 8-ounce can pineapple chunks, drained
1 red apple, unpeeled, cored, and diced (1 cup)
¼ cup nonfat salad dressing or reduced-fat mayonnaise
¼ cup low-fat sour cream (e.g., Friendship brand)
½ teaspoon grated lemon rind
1 tablespoon lemon juice
¼ cup dry-roasted soy nuts

In a medium-sized bowl, combine the cabbage and the fruit. In a small bowl, mix the salad dressing (or mayonnaise), sour cream, grated lemon rind, and lemon juice. Mix until smooth.

Lightly toss the dressing with the cabbage and the fruit. Cover and refrigerate for at least 30 minutes, if the time is available. Sprinkle with dry-roasted soy nuts and serve.

Serves four. Nutritional information per serving: 146 calories, 4 grams of fat, 3 grams of dietary fiber, 12 RE of vitamin A, 44 milligrams vitamin C.

Japanese Tofu Vegetable Salad

1 pound fresh green beans
2 cups broccoli flowerets (and stems if desired)
1½ cups sliced water chestnuts (canned)
1 cup canned or fresh bean sprouts
½ cup thinly sliced carrots
8-ounce bottle fat-free honey Dijon salad dressing
8 ounces firm tofu, well drained and cut into half-inch cubes

Steam or boil the fresh green beans for 3 to 4 minutes until *crisp but tender*. Drain and let cool. Combine the beans, broccoli, bean sprouts, and carrots and pour ¾ cup of the dressing over them. Cover and marinate approximately 30 minutes in the refrigerator. Pour remaining dressing over the tofu. Marinate both items in the refrigerator for 2 hours, time permitting. Drain both sets of ingredients from the dressing, arrange on a bed of lettuce or spinach, and serve with dressing on the side.

Serves three. Nutritional information per serving: 268 calories, 6 grams of fat, 11 grams of dietary fiber, 890 RE of vitamin A, 85 milligrams vitamin C.

Alternative homemade dressing for Japanese Tofu Vegetable Salad:

3 ounces rice vinegar
4 ounces orange juice
1 tablespoon honey

1 tablespoon low-sodium soy sauce
1 tablespoon sesame oil

Add ingredients together in a small bowl, mix with a wire whisk until honey is dissolved (about 5 minutes). Transfer to a screw-cap bottle or salad-dressing dispenser and shake vigorously before serving. Makes approximately 1 cup.

Mexican Zucchini

1 pound extrafirm tofu, crumbled
1 tablespoon olive oil
1 medium onion, diced
2 cloves finely minced garlic
3 cups chopped zucchini
½ cup tomato sauce
4 teaspoons low-sodium soy sauce
2 teaspoons dry chili powder
1 tablespoon chopped fresh basil (or 1 teaspoon dried)

To crumble the tofu, cut the 1-pound extrafirm cube into 5 or 6 large pieces. Pick up the pieces and push together in your hands; pieces should fall apart like feta cheese.

Sauté the onion and garlic in olive oil over medium heat for 2 to 4 minutes. Add the tofu and continue to stir for 3 more minutes. Add the zucchini and continue to sauté for 5 more minutes.

Add the remaining ingredients and bring the mix to a boil. Turn heat down and simmer over low heat for 3 minutes. May be served as a side dish or with baked corn tortilla chips.

Serves four. Nutritional information per serving (without chips): 169 calories, 6 grams of fat, 3 grams of dietary fiber, 104 RE of vitamin A, 16 milligrams vitamin C.

Chinese Coleslaw

1 tablespoon sesame seeds
¼ cup slivered almonds
1 head green cabbage, chopped (about 5 cups)
2 scallions with tops, finely chopped
¼ cup no-oil Italian salad dressing
2 teaspoons low-sodium soy sauce
¼ cup sugar
¼ cup white vinegar
½ cup grated radish (optional)

Preheat the oven to 350°F for 5 minutes. Place the slivered almonds and sesame seeds on a flat pizza pan and brown for about 3 to 4 minutes. Stir occasionally and do not overcook. Remove from heat and set aside. Turn off oven if not planning to use further.

In a medium-sized bowl, combine the cabbage and scallions. Chill in the refrigerator at least 30 minutes.

Combine the salad dressing, low-sodium soy sauce, sugar, and white vinegar in a small bowl, then blend with a wire whisk. At least twenty minutes before serving, toss together the almonds, sesame seeds, and cabbage mix. Pour the dressing over this mix and toss well. Garnish with grated radish, if you wish.

Serves six. Nutritional information per serving: 98 calories, 3 grams of fat, 2 grams of dietary fiber, 30 RE of vitamin A, 32 milligrams vitamin C.

Chinese Mixed Vegetables

1 Chinese green cabbage (about ½ pound bok choy)
1 tablespoon cooking oil
¼ teaspoon salt (optional)
6 ounces fresh asparagus
3 ripe medium tomatoes
5 ounces straw mushrooms
½ cup soup stock (low-sodium chicken broth, fat removed)
2 teaspoons low-sodium soy sauce
2 teaspoons water
2 teaspoons cornstarch
½ teaspoon sesame oil
2 teaspoons dry sherry or rice wine

Wash the cabbage, halving each stalk, and scald in boiling water. Remove and rinse in cold water; drain and set aside.

Heat the wok or large nonstick frying pan, add 1 tablespoon of cooking oil, and stir-fry the green cabbage. Season with ¼ teaspoon of salt, if desired, and stir until cooked. Remove and arrange on a platter.

Snip the asparagus into 1-inch pieces. Cook the asparagus and tomatoes in boiling water for 1 to 2 minutes. Remove and arrange the asparagus on the platter. Peel the tomatoes, if desired; otherwise, cut into halves or fourths and arrange on the platter. Scald the straw mushrooms in boiling water. Remove and set aside. Bring ½ cup soup stock and 2 teaspoons of soy sauce to a boil in the wok. Stir in the mushrooms and cook 1 minute. Lift mushrooms out and place on the platter.

Pour in 2 teaspoons of water and 2 teaspoons of cornstarch mixture to thicken the soup stock and soy sauce. Add the sesame oil and sherry/rice wine and stir continuously until thickened. Sprinkle over the vegetables on the platter and serve.

Serves six. Nutritional information per serving: 61 calories, 1–2 grams of fat, 2 grams of dietary fiber, 207 RE of vitamin A, 36 milligrams vitamin C.

Notes: As with other dishes, many different vegetables will easily adapt to this recipe. Try substituting green beans for the asparagus. To remove the fat from cans of chicken stock, place the can in the refrigerator about 30 minutes prior to using. The fat will congeal and then is easy to remove.

Broccoli-Flower Surprise

½ small firm cauliflower (2 cups)
2 cups chopped fresh broccoli
6–8 fresh plum tomatoes, chopped (2 cups)
½ cup chopped raw celery
½ cup diced carrots
½ cup diced zucchini
2 tablespoons sliced, pitted medium black olives
1 teaspoon fresh basil (if available) or ½ teaspoon dried
1 clove finely minced garlic
¼ teaspoon dried oregano
2 tablespoons grated Parmesan or Romano cheese

Heat about 1 inch of water in covered pot until it boils. If possible, use a steamer. Add the cauliflower and broccoli and simmer or steam about 10 to 15 minutes. Cook until vegetables are crisp but tender; do not overcook.

In a skillet or wok, mix the chopped tomatoes, celery, carrots, zucchini, and the olives. Add the basil, garlic, and oregano. Heat for 5 minutes, stirring occasionally.

Place the broccoli and cauliflower in a large bowl and cut into large chunks. Spoon the cooked vegetable mixture over the chunks and sprinkle with the grated cheese. Serve with a loaf of Italian bread.

Serves four. Nutritional information per serving: 94 calories, 2 grams of fat, 5 grams of dietary fiber, 678 RE of vitamin A, 97 milligrams vitamin C.

Notes: Try using green cauliflower, if available. Also go lightly on the olives—they contribute a hefty amount of fat when eaten in large amounts.

Carrot and Parsnip Puree

2 cups whole baby carrots, cut in ½-inch rounds
4 medium parsnips, sliced and diced (1½ cups)
6 ounces orange juice
½ teaspoon salt
½ teaspoon black pepper
1 tablespoon maple syrup
1½ teaspoons grated orange rind
½ cup brown raisins

Place the carrots and parsnips in a saucepan with boiling water to cover. Bring to a boil. Reduce the heat and simmer the vegetables, covered, for about 15 minutes or until tender. Drain.

Put the vegetables in a large bowl and add 2 ounces of orange juice, the salt, pepper, and maple syrup. Mash with a fork until smooth or place in an electric blender and blend until smooth.

Return the vegetable mixture to the saucepan with the rest of the orange juice for about 3 minutes, adding the grated orange rind and the raisins. Stir well and serve when heated.

Serves four. Nutritional information per serving: 176 calories, 1 gram of fat, 5 grams of dietary fiber, 1,531 RE of vitamin A, 38 milligrams vitamin C.

Tasty Sweet Turnips

½ teaspoon lemon juice
1 cup low-sodium chicken broth
2 teaspoons brown sugar
5 medium-sized turnips, peeled and cut into ⅛-inch slices
¼ cup brown raisins
2 tablespoons dry-roasted soy nuts
salt to taste

Stir the chicken broth, lemon juice, and brown sugar in a large frying pan. Heat until the mixture boils. Add the sliced turnips to the sauce and turn the flame down to simmer the turnips gently, covered, for about 15 minutes or until the slices are tender. Add a little more broth if necessary.

Mash the turnips until they are smooth and place them in a serving bowl. Mix in the raisins and the soy nuts, saving some of each to decorate on top.

Serves four. Nutritional information per serving: 89 calories, 1 gram of fat, 3 grams of dietary fiber, 1 RE of vitamin A, 15 milligrams vitamin C.

Tricolor Carrot Crunch

5 thin carrots, peeled and sliced in ½-inch rounds
1 cup celery, sliced on the diagonal in 1-inch pieces

2 teaspoons fresh lemon juice
½ teaspoon grated lemon rind
¼ teaspoon salt
⅛ teaspoon pepper
1 cup sliced red radishes
1 tablespoon chopped fresh dill (1 teaspoon dried)

Cook the sliced carrots and celery in a small amount of boiling water in a covered saucepan for about 8 to 10 minutes. The vegetables should be crisp but tender—*do not overcook.*

Drain and return the vegetables to the saucepan. Add lemon juice, grated lemon rind, salt, pepper, and sliced radishes. Heat quickly while stirring until all the vegetables are hot. Sprinkle with the chopped dill and serve.

Serves four. Nutritional information per serving: 47 calories, 0 grams of fat, 4 grams of dietary fiber, 1,919 RE of vitamin A, 13 milligrams vitamin C.

Carrots in Consommé

6 fresh carrots
1 cup of low-sodium chicken broth
1 tablespoon chopped fresh dill (or 1 teaspoon dried)

Peel and cut the carrots on the diagonal in 1-inch chunks. Place them in a small covered pot with 1 cup of chicken broth.

Steam the carrots covered in the liquid for 10 to 15 minutes, depending upon the size of the carrot pieces. The carrots should be crisp but tender—*do not overcook.*

Drain the liquid. Toss with the dill and serve.

Serves four. Nutritional information per serving: 51 calories, 0 grams of fat, 3 grams of dietary fiber, 3,038 RE of vitamin A, 11 milligrams vitamin C.

Stuffed Baked Apples

4 Rome Beauty baking apples (or any firm large apple)
6 tablespoons all-fruit jam (any flavor)
1½ cups pink lemonade or 1½ cups apple juice

Cut off a slice at the top of each apple. Then peel around the top to remove the apple skin one-third of the way down.

With a sharp knife, make a circle in the apple center and remove the core and seeds. Avoid making a hole in the bottom of the apple. Fill each apple with 1½ tablespoons of jam and place them in a Pyrex baking dish. Add the lemonade or apple juice to the baking dish.

Place the pan in a pre-heated 350°F oven for 45 minutes. After 20 minutes, spoon the liquid in the baking dish into the cavity of the apples and continue baking. To test if the apples are done, gently pierce one with a fork. If still hard, let them bake for another 5 to 7 minutes.

When finished, let the apples cool, then refrigerate.

Serves four. Nutritional information per serving: 186 calories, 1 gram of fat, 4 grams of dietary fiber, 6 RE of vitamin A, 7 milligrams vitamin C.

Karen's Vegetable Soup

3½ cups water
1 tablespoon chicken-flavored bouillon granules

1 can (14½ ounce) *no-salt-added* tomatoes, undrained and
    chopped
¼ cup diced green onions
1 tablespoon fresh basil (or 1 teaspoon dried)
1 teaspoon paprika
2 cloves minced garlic
¼ teaspoon salt (optional)
1 cup sliced carrots
2 cups chopped green cabbage
1 cup diced zucchini
1 cup diced, cooked white chicken meat (optional)
2 tablespoons Burgundy or other dry red wine

Combine the water, bouillon granules, tomatoes, onions, basil, paprika, garlic, and salt in a large pot. Bring to a boil. Cover, reduce heat, and simmer for 10 minutes. Add the carrots and cabbage; cover and simmer 10 more minutes. Add the zucchini, chicken, and wine; simmer uncovered an additional 8 minutes. Serve hot.

Serves six. Nutritional information per serving: 81 calories, 1 gram of fat, 2 grams of dietary fiber, 735 RE of vitamin A, 27 milligrams vitamin C.

Carrot and Bean Stew

12 ounces turkey sausage
2 cans (14–16 ounce) cooked beans (pinto, red kidney, or other
    varieties)
2 cups stewed tomatoes
2 cups sliced carrots
1 medium onion, chopped
1 cup sliced celery

1 potato with skin, diced
½ cup chopped fresh parsley
1 cup low-sodium chicken stock
2 bay leaves
2 teaspoons black pepper
1 teaspoon cayenne pepper
salt to taste
2 cloves finely minced garlic

Boil the turkey sausage for 15 minutes, piercing the skin in several places to allow the fat to drain from individual links. Remove from the liquid and cut into ½-inch pieces. Set aside.

Mix the cooked beans, stewed tomatoes, carrots, onion, celery, potato, parsley, and chicken stock in a large pot and bring to a boil. Add the bay leaves, black and cayenne pepper, salt, garlic, and sausage. Stir thoroughly. Add additional water as necessary.

Once boiling, simmer on low heat for at least 60 minutes. Serve with Italian bread.

Serves eight. Nutritional information per serving: 384 calories, 8 grams of fat, 9 grams of dietary fiber, 1,039 RE of vitamin A, 21 milligrams vitamin C.

Variations: This recipe is ideal for cooking overnight in a Crock-Pot. You may also add other beans to the recipe as desired.

Hearty Cabbage Soup

8 cups beef broth (use 4 beef bouillon cubes with 8 cups of boiling water)
2 medium Idaho potatoes, coarsely diced, with skin
1 sliced medium onion

3 carrots sliced (2 cups)
1 cup chopped canned tomatoes or stewed tomatoes
4 cups thinly sliced green cabbage
2 stalks sliced celery
2 tablespoons chopped curly parsley (fresh)
1 teaspoon oregano
1 cup frozen green peas

In a large pot, bring beef broth to a boil. Add the potatoes, onion, carrots, tomatoes, cabbage, celery, parsley, and oregano. Return to a boil. Then lower the heat and simmer, covering the pot for 30 to 40 minutes, until the vegetables are tender and *not* overcooked. Add 1 cup of frozen green peas and simmer for 3 minutes.

Serves six. Nutritional information per serving: 171 calories, 0 grams of fat, 7 grams of dietary fiber, 1,334 RE of vitamin A, 45 milligrams vitamin C.

Red Peppers and Pasta

4–6 red bell peppers
4 cups zucchini
½ cup green string beans, cut in ½-inch pieces
1 medium onion, coarsely chopped
1 teaspoon olive oil
½ cup water or nonfat chicken stock
4 cups chopped fresh tomatoes
3 ounces grated Romano cheese
1 pound of pasta (spinach or carrot linguini)
3 tablespoons fresh basil (3 teaspoons dried)
salt and pepper to taste

Cut the peppers in half lengthwise and remove the stems, seeds, and white pulp. Place cut edges facedown on a cookie sheet and bake for 15 minutes at 450–500°F. The skins should begin to get a bit dark; make sure they do not overcook at this point. Now place the cut peppers directly under the broiler and cook until the skin is blackened and raised above the surface. Be sure not to overcook the peppers; the underlying flesh should still be moist. When finished, place them in a covered dish (or paper bag) for 5 to 10 minutes. When cool, remove all skins from the peppers. Cut in ½-inch squares and set aside.

Place the zucchini, beans, onion, and olive oil in a large skillet and stir for 2 minutes over medium heat. Add the water (or stock), stir, and cover. Let cook over medium high heat for 10 minutes (until zucchini and beans begin to soften). Stir in the tomatoes and bring back to a low boil (about 5 minutes).

Prepare the pasta according to the directions on the package and place in a bowl. Pour the heated vegetables over the pasta and stir in the diced roasted peppers. Stir half of the Romano cheese into the bowl and add the fresh basil. Stir together and serve. Add Romano cheese, salt, and pepper as desired.

Serves four. Nutritional information per serving: 330 calories, 7 grams of fat, 6 grams of dietary fiber, 1,144 RE of vitamin A, 201 milligrams vitamin C.

Linguini Florentine

2 pounds fresh spinach, thoroughly washed
12 ounces uncooked linguini
2 teaspoons olive oil
2 ounces grated Parmesan cheese
½ teaspoon black pepper
1 tablespoon chopped walnuts

Remove the stems from the spinach and wash the leaves thoroughly. Tear the leaves into several large pieces. Cook the spinach covered in a large pot for about 4 minutes over low heat. *Do not add water.* Drain well; finely chop the leaves and set them aside.

Cook linguini according to the directions on the package, omitting the addition of salt and/or oil to the water. Drain. Combine the linguini and olive oil in a large bowl and toss gently. Add the spinach, Parmesan cheese, and pepper. Toss lightly and sprinkle with walnuts.

Serves four. Nutritional information per serving: 275 calories, 8 grams of fat, 7 grams of dietary fiber, 1,889 RE of vitamin A, 23 milligrams vitamin C.

Tofu Lasagna

12 ounces lasagna noodles
10 ounces cleaned spinach
1 tablespoon olive oil
1 medium onion, chopped
1 clove finely minced garlic
½ pound mushrooms
12 ounces firm tofu, mashed
4 ounces grated Parmesan or Romano cheese
2 beaten egg whites
2 tablespoons chopped parsley
1 tablespoon low-sodium soy sauce
½ teaspoon pepper
3 cups nonfat spaghetti sauce
½ cup part-skim-milk mozzarella cheese, grated

Cook the lasagna noodles according to the instructions on the package, drain, and set aside. Rinse, chop, and steam the spinach lightly, then set aside. Sauté the onion, garlic, and mushrooms in the olive oil for 2 to 4 minutes and set aside when finished.

In a large bowl, mix the tofu, Parmesan or Romano cheese, egg whites, parsley, soy sauce, and pepper. Add the sautéed vegetables and mix thoroughly.

Lightly coat the bottom of a glass eight-by-eleven baking dish with a nonstick oil spray. Place a row of lasagna noodles along the bottom. Build layers, alternating with noodles, tofu mixture, spaghetti sauce, spinach, and mozzarella cheese. The final layer should be spaghetti sauce.

Cover the dish with aluminum foil; bake in a preheated oven at 350°F for 40 minutes.

Serves six. Nutritional information per serving: 357 calories, 10 grams of fat, 5 grams of dietary fiber, 934 RE of vitamin A, 17 milligrams vitamin C.

Pizza Perfect

precooked pizza crusts (4 small or 1 large, Boboli brand)
1¼ cups nonfat spaghetti sauce (Healthy Choice)
½ cup crumbled extrafirm tofu
1 ounce sliced, pitted black olives
½ cup assorted chopped fresh vegetables (red or green pepper, zucchini, carrots, mushrooms, broccoli)
2 ounces part-skim-milk mozzarella cheese, shredded
1–2 ounces grated Romano or Parmesan cheese
¼ teaspoon dried oregano (optional)

Preheat oven to 450°F for 15 minutes.

Spread the pizza crusts with the pasta sauce. Next sprinkle the crumbled tofu, followed by black olives and chopped fresh vegetables. Then sprinkle the mozzarella and grated cheese evenly on all crusts, as well as oregano, if used.

Bake until the mozzarella cheese melts—about 10 minutes.

Serves four. Nutritional information per serving: 199 calories, 8 grams of fat, 3 grams of dietary fiber, 814 RE of vitamin A, 33 milligrams vitamin C.

Spaghetti with Meat Sauce

12 ounces extralean ground beef
2 cups nonfat spaghetti sauce
2 teaspoons dried oregano
½ pound pasta (spaghetti, linguini, ziti, etc.)
1 tablespoon chopped fresh parsley
grated Parmesan or Romano cheese (optional)

Sauté the ground beef over medium heat in a nonstick pan. Turn the meat frequently with a large plastic spoon or spatula until the beef is completely brown.

Thoroughly drain the liquid from the meat and then place the cooked meat on a couple of paper towels. Blot off all excess fat and liquid. Return the meat to the pan. Add the pasta sauce and oregano. Heat slowly, covered, until sauce begins to boil.

Cook the pasta according to the directions on the package and then pour the heated sauce over the drained pasta. Sprinkle the chopped parsley on top, as well as some grated Parmesan or Romano cheese if desired.

Serves four. Nutritional information per serving: 369 calories, 6–9 grams of fat, 3 grams of dietary fiber, 510 RE of vitamin A, 10 milligrams vitamin C.

Comments: We include this recipe to remind you that you can prepare ground beef in a breast-healthy manner.

Linguini Primavera

1 tablespoon olive oil
¼ cup chopped onions
2 cloves minced garlic
½ cup coarsely chopped green pepper
½ cup coarsely chopped red bell pepper
½ cup sliced carrots
2 cups fresh broccoli, cut up in bite-sized pieces
½ cup low-salt chicken stock (or 1 packet bouillon in ½ cup
    water)
1 pound linguini (try fresh spinach linguini)
1½ cups canned stewed tomatoes, chopped
½ teaspoon oregano (optional)
1 ounce grated Parmesan or Romano cheese

Lightly brown the onions and garlic in the olive oil, using a nonstick frying pan or wok (about 3 minutes). Add the peppers, carrots, and broccoli. Then add the chicken stock. Stir over heat for 2 minutes, then cover the pan and cook the vegetables until *crisp but tender*.

In the meantime, prepare the linguini according to the directions on the package. Heat the stewed tomatoes, adding oregano, in a separate pot for 3 minutes or until hot. Pour the crisp vegetables over the hot drained linguini and add the stewed tomatoes. Sprinkle with Parmesan or Romano cheese and toss lightly.

Serves four. Nutritional Information per serving: 253 calories, 6 grams of fat, 6 grams of dietary fiber, 786 RE of vitamin A, 97 milligrams vitamin C.

Variations: This dish allows for almost endless variety: You can add chopped cauliflower, green beans, chopped celery or zucchini, or fresh mushrooms. Have fun! Add whatever is in your refrigerator—you can't go wrong.

Italian-Style Chicken Cutlets

4 chicken breast cutlets (boned)
2 egg whites
¾ cup flavored bread crumbs
1½ tablespoons olive oil
6 ounces low-fat or nonfat marinara sauce (Healthy Choice)
1 teaspoon dried oregano
2 ounces part-skim-milk or nonfat mozzarella cheese, shredded
½ cup chopped fresh parsley

Preheat the oven to 350°F.

Dip the chicken cutlets in the beaten egg whites and then in the bread crumbs. Set aside.

Heat the olive oil in a nonstick skillet over a medium flame. Add the chicken breasts to the pan and cook on each side for 5 to 7 minutes, until lightly browned. Removed from pan and place on a paper towel to blot any excess oil. Place the cutlets in a single layer on a baking dish or square foil pan.

Spoon 3 tablespoons of marinara sauce on each piece of chicken and sprinkle oregano on top of the sauce. Top the cutlets with shredded mozzarella cheese and place in the oven. Bake for 15 to 20 minutes, until the chicken is hot and the cheese is melted. Top with chopped parsley.

Serves four. Nutritional information per serving: 304 calories, 8 grams of fat, 1 gram of dietary fiber, 107 RE of vitamin A, 9 milligrams vitamin C.

Chicken Sauté with Fresh Vegetables

4 chicken cutlets (1 pound), cut in thin strips (skinless and
    boneless)
1 tablespoon olive oil
10 ounces fresh brussels sprouts
1 medium onion, sliced
4 medium red-skinned potatoes (washed and unpeeled), cut in
    large chunks
4 carrots, cut in thick slices
1 cup low-sodium chicken broth (or bouillon cubes)
2 tablespoons chopped fresh dill and/or fresh parsley (2 teaspoons
    dried dill)
salt and pepper to taste

Lightly season the chicken with salt and pepper. Heat the olive oil
over medium heat and add the chicken to a large nonstick frying
pan with deep sides. Sauté uncovered until the chicken is lightly
browned (about 5 to 7 minutes each side). Drain and discard any
oil left in the pan.

Add the brussels sprouts, sliced onion, potatoes, carrots, and the
cup of chicken broth. Cover the chicken and vegetables and simmer
for a half hour until tender. *Do not overcook.* Sprinkle with chopped
dill or chopped parsley.

Serves four. Nutritional information per serving: 468 calories, 9
grams of fat, 9 grams of dietary fiber, 2,082 RE of vitamin A, 83
milligrams vitamin C.

Turkey Cutlets with Spicy Fruit Sauce

1¼ cups canned unsweetened pineapple juice
¼ cup golden raisins
¼ cup dried apricots
½ teaspoon cayenne pepper
2 cloves finely minced garlic
4 4-ounce turkey breast cutlets
2 ounces all-fruit apricot jam
1 teaspoon cornstarch
1 scallion

Combine the pineapple juice, raisins, apricots, cayenne pepper, and garlic in a large nonstick skillet. Bring to a boil. Add the turkey cutlets. Cover the pan, reduce the heat, and simmer for 10 to 12 minutes or until the turkey is done.

Remove the turkey and keep warm in the oven.

Bring the cooking liquid to a boil. Cook 5 to 7 minutes or until reduced to about ¾ cup. Stir occasionally. Combine the jam and cornstarch. Stir into cooking liquid and cook for 1 minute until thickened.

Spoon 3 tablespoons over each turkey cutlet and garnish with chopped scallion or onion strips and fresh parsley as desired.

Serves four. Nutritional information per serving: 321 calories, 3 grams of fat, 2 grams of dietary fiber, 155 RE of vitamin A, 9 milligrams vitamin C.

Chicken and Vegetable Salad

4 ounces skinless, boneless chicken breast
1–2 heads red-leaf lettuce (8 cups)
1 wedge red cabbage, finely sliced (about 1 cup)
4 ounces pitted black olives
4-ounce package feta cheese
2–3 large carrots, washed and unpeeled, sliced (1 cup)
3 plum tomatoes
2 tablespoons chopped walnuts
8 ounces fat-free honey Dijon salad dressing
melba toast

Cut the chicken into long, thin strips and place in a pot of boiling water for approximately 15 minutes. When done, transfer to a bowl of ice water to cool quickly (5 minutes). In the meantime, wash the lettuce and drain. Chop lettuce into bite-size pieces and transfer to a large salad bowl. Slice the red cabbage into thin pieces, using a food processor or large knife. Then pull apart into thin shreds and transfer to the bowl. Drain and slice olives, and place in the bowl. Crumble or dice the feta cheese and place in the bowl. Place slivered carrots into the bowl. Dice the plum tomatoes and add them and the walnuts to the salad bowl. When the chicken is cool, cut the slivers into small bite-size pieces and add to the bowl.

Mix salad thoroughly. Add salad dressing and serve with melba toast on the side.

Serves eight. Nutritional information per serving: 214 calories, 6 grams of fat, 4 grams of dietary fiber, 579 RE of vitamin A, 23 milligrams vitamin C.

Variations: This salad can be the basis for endless variations: Try adding watercress, arugula, dandelion greens, kale, or fresh parsley. The tastes of these greens mix perfectly.

Oriental Chicken Platter

1 cup brown rice
4 small chicken cutlets (thin-sliced)
5 tablespoons flour
2 tablespoons canola oil
½ cup firm tofu, cubed
¾ cup red and green pepper strips
1 cup broccoli flowerets
1 cup cauliflower pieces
½ cup sliced fresh mushrooms
½ cup canned water chestnuts, sliced
½ cup low-sodium soy sauce
1 cup chicken broth (or 2 bouillon cubes in a cup of hot water)
2 tablespoons dry-roasted soy nuts

Start making the brown rice right away, following the directions on the package. It will require about 30 to 50 minutes, depending upon the brand. If your time is limited, quick-cooking brown rice is also available.

Cut the chicken cutlets into 2-inch pieces and dip them in a plate with the flour. Heat the oil in a large skillet or wok and sauté the chicken pieces along with the tofu until they are all lightly browned. Take the chicken and tofu out with a slotted spoon and set aside.

Add the vegetables to the pan and sprinkle the soy sauce over them. Sauté quickly over high heat for about 3 to 5 minutes. Add the chicken broth and the cooked rice. Simmer the chicken and tofu with the vegetables and rice for another 5 minutes until hot. Sprinkle the chopped soy nuts on top.

Serves four. Nutritional information per serving: 354 calories, 12 grams of fat, 4 grams of dietary fiber, 144 RE of vitamin A, 73 milligrams vitamin C.

Chicken with Broccoli

1 cup brown rice
2 cups broccoli flowerets (include stems if desired)
2 teaspoons cornstarch
¼ teaspoon black pepper
½ cup low-sodium chicken broth (can be made with bouillon
    cubes)
1 tablespoon olive oil
1 clove garlic, peeled and diced
1 whole chicken breast, skinned, boned, and cut into ½-inch
    cubes
½ cup sliced water chestnuts
½ cup sliced carrots

Cook the brown rice according to the directions on the package. Do this before beginning to prepare the rest of the recipe.

Simmer the broccoli in boiling water (or use a vegetable steamer) for 3 to 4 minutes. Do not overcook; broccoli should still be deep green and crisp.

Mix the cornstarch, pepper, and chicken broth. Stir and set aside.

Pour the oil into a frying pan or hot wok and turn heat to medium high. When the oil is hot, sauté the garlic briefly and then add the chicken. Cook the chicken until the pieces are lightly browned, turning frequently.

Add the broccoli to the pan and stir. Cover the pan or wok, lower the heat, and cook for 3 minutes. Add the water chestnuts and carrots. Stir well to mix with the chicken and broccoli. Stir the cornstarch-broth mix and pour over the chicken and vegetables. Continue to stir over low heat until sauce thickens.

Serves two. Nutritional information per serving: 393 calories, 10 grams of fat, 7 grams of dietary fiber, 1,099 RE of vitamin A, 84 milligrams vitamin C.

Variations: Try about ½ teaspoon of freshly grated ginger root. Another delightful addition is a few dry-roasted unsalted peanuts or soy nuts.

Sautéed Tofu and Vegetables

1 teaspoon roasted sesame oil
1 cup onions sliced into half-moons
1 cup fresh sweet corn, removed from the cob (2 ears)
1 cup red cabbage, sliced into ½-inch chunks
1 pound extrafirm tofu, crumbled by hand
1 tablespoon soy sauce
½ cup diced sweet red peppers
1 cup brown rice

Heat the sesame oil in a wok or large skillet. Sauté the onions over medium heat until golden brown (about 5 minutes). Stir in the corn and cabbage. Sprinkle the crumbled tofu into the mixture, stirring frequently. Add the soy sauce.

Reduce heat to low, and cook for a few more minutes. *Do not overcook*—keep the vegetables crispy. Remove and place in serving bowl. Garnish with diced red pepper. Serve with brown rice, cooked according to the directions on the package.

Serves four. Nutritional information per serving: 244 calories, 11 grams of fat, 4 grams of dietary fiber, 95 RE of vitamin A, 40 milligrams vitamin C.

Tofu Rancheros

1 teaspoon roasted sesame oil
1 teaspoon vegetable oil (peanut or olive)
1 leek, diced
2 carrots, diced
3 ears corn, kernels cut off cob (about 1 cup)
spices and herbs (optional): pinch cumin, ¼–½ teaspoon cayenne
    pepper, teaspoon chopped cilantro
½ pound firm tofu, diced
½ cup salsa
1 tablespoon miso powder (if available)
1 tablespoon arrowroot or cornstarch, dissolved in 1 cup water
⅓ cup chopped scallions

Heat the oil in a wok or skillet and sauté diced vegetables for 3 to 5 minutes. Add the herbs and spices as desired. Stir in the diced tofu and continue to stir over low heat for 3 minutes.

Mix the salsa, miso, and dissolved arrowroot or cornstarch in water in a small bowl. Add this mixture to the wok or skillet, raise heat, and stir until sauce becomes thick and shiny. Simmer on low heat for 5 minutes. When finished, add chopped scallions and serve.

Serves four. Nutritional information per serving: 221 calories, 7 grams of fat, 6 grams of dietary fiber, 1,121 RE of vitamin A, 19 milligrams vitamin C.

Variations: Serve with nonfat tortilla chips or baked flour tortillas.

Sweet-and-Sour Veggies

1 teaspoon cornstarch
2 tablespoons water
16-ounce can pineapple chunks (in the juice)
¼ cup water
1 tablespoon rice vinegar
1 teaspoon brown sugar
¼–½ teaspoon grated ginger (optional)
dash of black pepper
¼ teaspoon salt (optional)
1 pound firm tofu, cut into ½-inch cubes
2 tablespoons olive oil
1 onion, chopped
1 large carrot, sliced into thin strips
1 cup thinly sliced green, red, and/or yellow peppers
½ cup diced celery
1 cup brown rice or package of Oriental (nonfried) lo mein noo-
      dles

Dissolve the cornstarch in 2 tablespoons of water. Drain the pineapple and save the juice. Mix ¼ cup water, ¼ cup pineapple juice,
vinegar, sugar, ginger, black pepper, and salt. Set aside.

In a large skillet or wok, sauté tofu cubes over medium heat in 1
tablespoon of olive oil until brown. Remove with a slotted spoon
and set aside. Add the additional 1 tablespoon of oil and sauté the
onion until golden brown (4 to 5 minutes). Add the carrots, peppers
and celery and continue to sauté over medium heat for an additional
2 to 3 minutes. Do not overcook.

Add tofu to the sautéed vegetables in the wok and mix thoroughly.
Add pineapple chunks, together with the liquid/spice mixture and
stir. Add the cornstarch and stir over medium high heat until the
mixture thickens. Serve alone or over brown rice or noodles.

Serves four. Nutritional information per serving: 314 calories, 10 grams of fat, 4 grams of dietary fiber, 563 RE of vitamin A, 55 milligrams vitamin C.

Ratatouille with Tofu

1 tablespoon olive oil
1–2 medium onions, diced (1 cup)
2 cloves finely minced garlic
½ pound plum tomatoes, diced
½ pound firm tofu, cut into ½-inch cubes
1 teaspoon fresh basil (or ½ teaspoon dried)
¼ teaspoon oregano
1 stalk celery, sliced
1–2 zucchini, sliced (1½ cups)
1 sweet red bell pepper, cut into strips
2 cups eggplant, peeled and cubed
½ cup mushrooms

Heat olive oil in a large skillet or wok. Sauté the onion and garlic until onion is tender and golden brown (about 4 to 5 minutes). While the heat is still high, add the tomatoes, tofu, basil, and oregano. Turn the heat to low and add the celery, zucchini, red pepper, eggplant, and mushrooms. Cover the skillet and simmer on low heat for 30 minutes. Serve hot or cold. May be served with Italian bread.

Serves four. Nutritional information per serving: 289 calories, 8 grams of fat, 5 grams of dietary fiber, 205 RE of vitamin A, 56 milligrams vitamin C.

French Country Stew

vegetable-oil spray
1 pound extrafirm tofu
**herbs (optional): ½ teaspoon dried sage, ½ teaspoon dried thyme,
  1 bay leaf, ½ teaspoon dried parsley**
½ cup onion, sliced
1 medium carrot, cut into ½-inch slices
½ cup string beans
1 medium sweet potato or yam, cut into ¾-inch slices
1½ cups water
½ teaspoon salt (optional)
3 tablespoons wheat flour
2 cloves finely minced garlic
¼ teaspoon Tabasco sauce
1 tablespoon low-sodium soy sauce
1 package frozen peas (12 ounces)

Spray a large skillet or wok with cooking oil, bring to medium heat, and brown the tofu (about 5 minutes). Set aside.

In a 3-quart pot, combine the herbs, onions, carrot, string beans, sweet potato, 1 cup of water, and salt. Bring to a boil. Then turn down the heat and simmer for 20 minutes or until the vegetables are crisp but tender. Add the flour, garlic, Tabasco sauce, soy sauce, and remaining ½ cup of water to the pot, return to a boil, and continue to cook over low heat for about 5 more minutes.

Add the peas and tofu and cook an additional 5 minutes. Serve when finished.

Serves four. Nutritional information per serving: 233 calories, 3 grams of fat, 7 grams of dietary fiber, 1,194 RE of vitamin A, 20 milligrams vitamin C.

Tangy Szechuan Broccoli and Rice

1 cup brown rice
1 tablespoon low-sodium soy sauce
1 tablespoon rice vinegar
1 teaspoon sugar
1 tablespoon sesame seeds
1½ tablespoons canola oil
½ teaspoon minced ginger root
2 cloves garlic, peeled and diced
5 cups coarsely chopped broccoli flowerets and stems

Start the brown rice according to the directions. This may require up to 50 minutes, so it should be started first.

Combine the soy sauce, rice vinegar, and sugar in a small bowl; set aside. Heat a large skillet or wok over medium heat. Add the sesame seeds and cook 1 minute or until browned. Remove the seeds and set aside.

Add oil, ginger, and garlic to the skillet or wok on high heat and stir-fry for 30 seconds. Add the broccoli and stir-fry for 1 minute. Add the soy sauce mixture and stir well. Cover and cook for 2 minutes or until broccoli is crisp but tender. Sprinkle with the sesame seeds. Serve on a platter of brown rice.

Serves four. Nutritional information per serving: 196 calories, 7 grams of fat, 5 grams of dietary fiber, 170 RE of vitamin A, 103 milligrams vitamin C.

Variations: Different types of nuts easily fit in this recipe in place of the sesame seeds. Try adding chopped walnuts or dry-roasted soy nuts (¼ cup). But go lightly with the nuts: They add quite a bit of fat to the recipe.

Tofu Stir-Fry with Wine

½ cup sake or white cooking wine
3 tablespoons low-sodium soy sauce
2 teaspoons ginger juice (optional)
2 cloves minced garlic
12 ounces extrafirm tofu, cut into ½-inch cubes
1½ tablespoons sesame oil
1 medium onion, chopped (½ cup)
1 red pepper, sliced and diced
2 cups sliced Chinese cabbage (bok choy) (substitute broccoli if
      bok choy is unavailable)
1 package (8 ounces) frozen snow peas
1 cup canned pineapple chunks, drained
2 tablespoons dry-roasted soy nuts or slivered almonds
1 cup brown rice

In a wok or heavy skillet, bring wine, soy sauce, and garlic to a
boil. Add the tofu cubes, cover, and simmer for 5 minutes on a low
flame. Remove the tofu and liquid from the pan and set aside.

Heat the sesame oil, and stir-fry the vegetables over medium high
heat for 3 to 5 minutes. Stir in the remaining broth and tofu, add
the pineapple and the nuts, and heat over medium heat for an
additional 2 minutes. Serve over a bed of brown rice.

Serves four. Nutritional information per serving: 350 calories, 10
grams of fat, 7 grams of dietary fiber, 201 RE of vitamin A, 78
milligrams vitamin C.

Vegetable Omelet

6 egg whites
⅓ cup chopped fresh tomatoes
½ cup chopped red and green pepper
salt and pepper to taste
2 tablespoons chopped parsley
2 tablespoons chopped carrots
1½ tablespoons canola oil
½ teaspoon oregano

Break the eggs into a medium-sized bowl and discard the yolks. Beat the egg whites thoroughly. Combine the chopped vegetables in a small dish and lightly season with salt and pepper to taste.

Heat the oil in a 10-inch nonstick frying pan and distribute over the entire surface of the pan. Pour in the beaten egg whites and let cook over a medium flame until the omelet is almost set. Do not stir.

Add the chopped vegetables evenly over the omelet and sprinkle on the oregano. Let the omelet cook until the vegetable-egg mixture is no longer runny.

Use a thin spatula to loosen the omelet from the bottom and sides of the pan. Flip it over into a half-moon and remove from the pan. Cut in half and serve with toast.

Serves two. Nutritional information per serving: 163 calories, 10 grams of fat, 2 grams of dietary fiber, 426 RE of vitamin A, 100 milligrams vitamin C.

Salmon Salad

1 7½-ounce can red salmon
1 teaspoon lemon juice
1 teaspoon grated onion
¼ cup shredded carrots
¼ cup diced radish
¼ cup chopped celery
1 tablespoon nonfat sour cream
1 tablespoon reduced-fat mayonnaise or salad dressing
4–6 leaves red-leaf lettuce
6 slices whole-wheat bread

Drain the canned salmon. Remove any skin and bones and chop well. Add the grated onions and the chopped vegetables.

Combine the sour cream, salad dressing, and lemon juice. Mix with the chopped salmon and vegetables. Chill in the refrigerator. Serve on toasted whole-wheat or other bread.

Serves three. Nutritional information per serving: 248 calories, 9 grams of fat, 6 grams of dietary fiber, 301 RE of vitamin A, 5 milligrams vitamin C.

Skinny French Toast

4 teaspoons all-fruit jam
4 slices whole-wheat bread
2 egg whites
1 egg yolk
¼ cup 1% milk
½ teaspoon brown sugar
¼ teaspoon ground cinnamon
¼ teaspoon ground nutmeg
vegetable-oil spray

Thoroughly beat the egg whites and the yolk. Add the milk, sugar, cinnamon, and nutmeg to the egg mixture. Let the bread soak in the eggs on both sides.

Spray a non-stick pan (before heating) for 2–3 seconds with the vegetable-oil spray. Heat the pan to cooking temperature and add the egg-coated bread. Cook on both sides until lightly browned.

Serve with either all-fruit jam or maple syrup.

Serves two. Nutritional information per serving: 227 calories, 5 grams of fat, 4 grams of dietary fiber, 42 RE of vitamin A, 1 milligram vitamin C.

REFERENCES

Chapter One

Cancer Control Objectives for the Nation: 1985–2000, vol. 68. Sondik, E. Washington, D.C.: NCI Monographs, 1986.

Review of evidence on the early detection and treatment of breast cancer. Morrison, A. S. *Cancer* 64(1989):2651–2656.

Using mammography for cancer control: an unrealized potential. Howard, J. CA-A *Cancer Journal for Clinicians* 37(1987):33–48.

Cancer prevention: recent progress and future opportunities. Weinstein, I. B. *Cancer Research* 51, suppl. (1991):5080s–5085s.

Faulty math heightens fears of breast cancer. Blakeslee, S. *The New York Times*, March 15, 1992, E1.

Refiguring the odds: what's a woman's real chance of suffering breast cancer? Fackelmann, K. A. *Science News*, 144(1993):76–77.

Cancer statistics, 1992. Boring, C. C., T. S. Squires, and T. Tong. CA-A *Cancer Journal for Clinicians* 42(1992):19–35.

Breast cancer (first of three parts). Harris, J. R., M. E. Lippman, U. Veronesi, et al. *New England Journal of Medicine* 327 (1992):319–326.

Mammography screening and increased incidence of breast cancer in Wisconsin. Lantz, P. M., P. L. Remington, and P. A. Newcomb. *Journal of the National Cancer Institute* 83(1991):1540–1546.

The control of breast cancer. A World Health Organization perspective. Koroltchouk, V., K. Stanley, and J. Stjernsward. *Cancer* 65(1990): 2803–2810.

Insights into fruit and vegetable consumption: a summary of recent findings for planning the 5-a-Day program. NCI Office of Cancer Communications. National Institutes of Health, June 8, 1992.

Fruit, vegetables, and cancer prevention: a review of the epidemiological evidence. Block, G., B. Patterson, and A. Subar. *Nutrition and Cancer*, 18(1992):1–29.

Cigarette smoking in women with cancers of the breast and reproductive organs. Baron, J. A., T. Byers, E. R. Greenberg, et al. *Journal of the National Cancer Institute* 77(1986):677–680.

Increased 2-hydroxylation of estradiol as a possible mechanism for the antiestrogenic effect of cigarette smoking. Michnovicz, J. J., R. J. Hershcopf, H. Naganuma, et al. *New England Journal of Medicine* 315(1986):1305–1309.

Increased urinary catechol estrogen excretion in female smokers. Michnovicz, J. J., H. Naganuma, R. J. Hershcopf, et al. *Steroids* 52(1988):69–83.

Radiometric analysis of biological oxidations in man: sex differences in estradiol metabolism. Fishman, J., H. L. Bradlow, J. Schneider, et al. *Proceedings of the National Academy of Science, USA*, 77(1980):4957–4960.

Agreements signed to test foods for cancer prevention. Reynolds, T. *Journal of the National Cancer Institute* 83(1991):1050–1052.

Designer foods. Fackelmann, K. A. *Nutrition Action Health Letter*, 18(1991):1–7.

The dietary fat-breast cancer hypothesis is alive. Schatzkin, A., P. Greenwald, D. P. Byar, et al. *Journal of the American Medical Association* 261(1989):3284–3287.

Chapter Two

Breast cancer (second of three parts). Harris, J. R., M. E. Lippman, U. Veronesi, et al. *New England Journal of Medicine* 327(1992):389–398.

Mutation and cancer: a model for human carcinogenesis. Moolgavkar, S. H. and A. G. Knudson. *Journal of the National Cancer Institute* 66(1981):1037–1052.

Increased cell division as a cause of human cancer. Preston-Martin, S., M. C. Pike, R. K. Ross, et al. *Cancer Research* 50(1990):7415–7421.

Breast cancer (third of three parts). Harris, J. R., M. E. Lippman, U. Veronesi, et al. *New England Journal of Medicine* 327(1992):473–480.

Chemical carcinogenesis: Too many rodent carcinogens. Ames, B. N. and L. S. Gold. *Proceedings of the National Academy of Science, USA* 87(1990):7772–7776.

Hormonal chemoprevention of cancer in women. Henderson, B. E., R. K. Ross, and M. C. Pike. *Science* 259(1993):633–638.

A prospective study of the development of breast cancer in 16,692 women with benign breast disease. Carter, C. L., D. K. Corle, M. S. Micozzi, et al. *American Journal of Epidemiology* 128(1988):467–477.

The epidemiology of benign breast disease. Ernster, V. L. *Epidemiologic Reviews* 3(1981):184–202.

Evaluation, diagnosis, and treatment of the fibrocystic breast. Marchant, D. J. *Modern Medicine* 55(1987):42–50.

Ductal carcinoma in situ (intraductal carcinoma) of the breast. Schnitt, S. J., W. Silen, N. L. Sadowsky, et al. *New England Journal of Medicine* 318(1988):898–902.

Refiguring the odds: what's a woman's real chance of suffering breast cancer? Fackelmann, K. A. *Science News* 144(1993):76–77.

Breast cancer (first of three parts). Harris, J. R., M. E. Lippman, U. Veronesi, et al. *New England Journal of Medicine* 327(1992):319–326.

Etiology of human breast cancer: a review. MacMahon, B., P. Cole, and J. Brown. *Journal of the National Cancer Institute* 50(1973):21–42.

The international variation in breast cancer rates: an epidemiological assessment. Henderson, B. E. and L. Bernstein. *Breast Cancer Research and Treatment* 18, suppl (1991):S11–S17.

Breast cancer family history as a risk factor for early onset breast cancer. Lynch, H. T., P. Watson, T. Conway, et al. *Breast Cancer Research and Treatment* 11(1988):263–267.

Clinical/genetic features in hereditary breast cancer. Lynch, H. T., P. Watson, T. A. Conway, et al. Breast Cancer Research and Treatment 15(1990):63–71.

Breast cancer risks in relatives of male breast cancer patients. Anderson, D. E. and M. D. Badzioch. Journal of the National Cancer Institute 84(1992):1114–1117.

Risk for breast cancer development determined by mammographic parenchymal pattern. Wolfe, J. N. Cancer 37(1976):2486–2492.

Nonpalpable, probably benign breast lesions: follow-up strategies after initial detection on mammography. Adler, D. D., M. A. Helvie, and D. M. Ikeda. American Journal of Radiology 155(1990):1195–1201.

Prospective study of relative weight, height, and risk of breast cancer. London, S. J., G. A. Colditz, M. J. Stampfer, et al. Journal of the American Medical Association 262(1989):2853–2858.

Body size and breast cancer risk assessed in women participating in the breast cancer detection demonstration project. Swanson, C. A., L. A. Brinton, P. R. Taylor, et al. American Journal of Epidemiology 130(1989):1133–1141.

Oral contraceptives and breast cancer. Thomas, D. B. Journal of the National Cancer Institute 85(1993):359–364.

A meta-analysis of the effect of estrogen replacement therapy on the risk of breast cancer. Steinberg, K. K., S. B. Thacker, S. J. Smith, et al. Journal of the American Medical Association 265(1991):1985–1990.

Alcohol and breast cancer risk—putting the controversy into perspective. Steinberg, J. and P. J. Goodwin. Breast Cancer Research and Treatment 19(1991):221–231.

Blood levels of organochlorine residues and risk of breast cancer. Wolff, M. S., P. G. Toniolo, E. W. Lee, et al. Journal of the National Cancer Institute 85(1993):648–652.

Environmental cancer risk factors. A review. Tomatis, L. Acta Oncologica 27, fasc. 5(1988):465–472.

Lower lifetime occurrence of breast cancer and cancers of the reproductive system among former college athletes. Frisch, R. E., G. Wyshak, J. Witschi, et al. International Journal of Fertility 32(1987):217–225.

Lower prevalence of breast cancers of the reproductive system among former college athletes compared to non-athletes. Frisch, R. E., G. Wyshak, N. L. Albright, et al. British Journal of Cancer 52(1985):885–891.

Estimate of breast cancer risk reduction with weight loss. Schapira, D. V., N. B. Kumar, and G. H. Lyman. *Cancer* 67(1991):2622–2625.

Upper-body fat distribution and endometrial cancer risk. Schapira, D. V., N. B. Kumar, G. H. Lyman, et al. *Journal of the American Medical Association* 266(1991):1808–1811.

The causes of cancer: quantitative estimates of avoidable risks of cancer in the United States today. Doll, R. and R. Peto. *Journal of the National Cancer Institute* 66(1981):1191–1308.

The lessons of life: keynote address to the Nutrition and Cancer Conference. Doll, R. *Cancer Research* 52, suppl (1992):2024s–2029s.

Chapter Three

Breast cancer in multi-ethnic populations: the Hawaii perspective. Goodman, M. J. *Breast Cancer Research and Treatment* 18, suppl (1991):S5–S9.

Diet and cancer. Cohen, L. A. *Scientific American* 257(1987):42–50.

The control of breast cancer. A World Health Organization perspective. Koroltchouk, V., K. Stanley, and J. Stjernsward. *Cancer* 65(1990): 2803–2810.

Dietary fat and mammary cancer. Carroll, K. K., E. B. Gammal, and E. R. Plunkett. *Canadian Medical Association Journal* 98(1968):590–594.

Fat and cancer. Carroll, K. K., L. M. Braden, J. A. Bell, et al. *Cancer* 58(1986):1818–1825.

Studies of Japanese migrants. I. Mortality from cancer and other diseases among Japanese in the United States. Haenszel, L. and M. Kurihara. *Journal of the National Cancer Institute* 40(1968):43–49.

Cancer mortality among the Polish-born in the United States. Staszewski, J. and W. Haenszel. *Journal of the National Cancer Institute* 35(1965):291–297.

Cancer mortality in 1970–1972 among Polish-born migrants to England and Wales. Adelstein, A. M., J. Staszewski, and C. S. Muir. *British Journal of Cancer* 40(1979):464–475.

Implications of recent Australian epidemiological studies for cancer prevention through dietary change. MacLennan, R., *Recent Progress in Research on Nutrition and Cancer*, eds. Mettlin, C. J. and K. Aoki. New York: Wiley-Liss, Inc., 1990, 35–44.

Europe: as many cancers as cuisines. Balter, M. *Science* 254(1991): 1114–1115.

A case-control study of breast cancer in Tianjin, China. Wang, Q.-S., R. K. Ross, M. C. Yu, et al. *Cancer Epidemiology, Biomarkers & Prevention* 1(1992):435–439.

Changing patterns of cancer and diet in Japan. Tominaga, S., and I. Kato. *Recent Progress in Research on Nutrition and Cancer*, eds. Mettlin, C. J. and K. Aoki. New York: Wiley-Liss, Inc. (1990), 1–10.

Methodology and evaluation of dietary factors in Japan. Y. Ohno. *Recent Progress in Research on Nutrition and Cancer*, eds. Mettlin, C. J. and K. Aoki. New York: Wiley-Liss, Inc., 1990, 11–20.

Rice farmers dig in: to them, the land is sacred. Pollack, A. *The New York Times*, February 18, 1993, A6.

Cancer patterns in Japan. T. Hirayama. *Origins of Human Cancer*, eds. Hiatt, H. H., J. D. Watson, and J. A. Winston. Cold Spring Harbor, New York: Cold Spring Harbor Laboratory, 1977, 69–71.

Chapter Four

The genesis and growth of tumors. III. Effects of a high-fat diet. Tannenbaum, A. *Cancer Research* 2(1942):468–475.

Relationship between dietary fat and experimental mammary tumorigenesis: a review and critique. Welsch, C. W. *Cancer Research* 52, suppl (1992):2040s–2048s.

Dietary factors and risk of breast cancer: combined analysis of 12 case-control studies. Howe, G. R., T. Hirohata, T. G. Hislop, et al. *Journal of the National Cancer Institute* 82(1990):561–569.

Dietary fat and fiber in relation to risk of breast cancer. Willett, W. C., D. J. Hunter, M. J. Stampfer, et al. *Journal of the American Medical Association* 268(1992):2037–2044.

What are people really eating? The relation between energy intake derived from estimated diet records and intake determined to maintain body weight. Mertz, W., J. C. Tsui, J. T. Judd, et al. *American Journal of Clinical Nutrition* 54(1991):291–295.

Discrepancy between self-reported and actual caloric intake and exercise in obese subjects. Lichtman, S. W., K. Pisarska, E. R. Berman, et al. *New England Journal of Medicine* 327(1992):1893–1898.

Feasibility of a randomized trial of a low-fat diet for the prevention of breast cancer: dietary compliance in the Women's Health Trial Vanguard Study. Henderson, M. M., L. H. Kushi, and D. J. Thompson. *Preventive Medicine* 19(1990):115–133.

Role of intervention trials in research on nutrition and cancer. Henderson, M. M. *Cancer Research* 52, suppl (1992):2030s–2034s.

Results of a randomized feasibility study of a low-fat diet. Insull, W., M. M. Henderson, and R. L. Prentice. *Archives of Internal Medicine* 150(1990):421–427.

Dietary fat reduction and plasma estradiol concentration in healthy post-menopausal women. Prentice, R., D. Thompson, C. Clifford, et al. *Journal of the National Cancer Institute* 82(1990):129–134.

How women's adopted low-fat diets affect their husbands. Shattuck, A. L., E. White, and A. R. Kristal. *American Journal of Public Health* 82(1992):1244–1250.

Maintenance of a low-fat diet: follow-up of the Women's Health Trial. White, E., A. L. Shattuck, A. R. Kristal, et al. *Cancer Epidemiology, Biomarkers & Prevention* 1(1992):315–323.

Low-fat diet trial set to take off. Smigel, K. *Journal of the National Cancer Institute* 82(1990):1736–1737.

Third strike for NCI breast cancer study. Marshall, E. *Science* 250(1990):1503–1504.

Current approaches to breast cancer prevention. Henderson, M. *Science* 259(1993):630–632.

NIH unveils plan for women's health project. Palca, J. *Science* 254(1991):792–793.

Chapter Five

Physiological effects of cabbage with reference to its potential as a dietary cancer-inhibitor and its use in ancient medicine. Albert-Puleo, M. *Journal of Ethnopharmacology* 9(1983):261–272.

Vegetables, fruit, and cancer. I. Epidemiology. Steinmetz, K. A. and J. D. Potter. *Cancer Causes and Control* 2(1991):325–357.

Vegetables, fruit, and cancer. II. Mechanisms. Steinmetz, K. A. and J. D. Potter. *Cancer Causes and Control* 2(1991):427–442.

Fruit, vegetables, and cancer prevention: a review of the epidemiological evidence. Block, G., B. Patterson, and A. Subar. *Nutrition and Cancer* 18(1992):1–29.

Inhibition of carcinogenesis by minor dietary constituents. Wattenberg, L. W. *Cancer Research* 52, suppl (1992):2085s–2091s.

Dietary pesticides (99.99% all natural). Ames, B. N., M. Profet, and L. S. Gold. *Proceedings of the National Academy of Science, USA* 87(1990):7777–7781.

The organization and function of NAPRALERT. Beecher, C. Wm. W., and N. R. Farnsworth. *Progress on Terrestrial and Marine Natural Products of Medicinal and Biological Interest*, eds. Pezzuto, J. M., A. D. Kinghorn, H. H. S. Fong, and G. A. Cordell. Austin, Texas: American Botanical Council, 1991, 146–153.

After 4,000 years, medical science considers garlic. Brody, J. E. *The New York Times*, September 4, 1990, C1.

Scientists seeking possible wonder drugs in tea. Brody, J. E. *The New York Times*, March 14, 1991, C8.

Chapter Six

On the treatment of inoperable cases of carcinoma of the mamma: suggestions for a new method of treatment with illustrative cases. Beatson, G. T. *Lancet* 2(1896):104–107.

The Dread Disease. Patterson, J. T. Cambridge: Harvard University Press, 1987.

Oestrogens and breast cancer. Miller, W. R. *British Medical Bulletin* 47(1990):470–483.

The role of endogenous estrogen excess in human breast cancer. Zumoff, B. *Anticancer Research* 1(1981):39–44.

Abnormal oxidative metabolism of estradiol in women with breast cancer.

Schneider, J., D. Kinne, A. Fracchia, et al. *Proceedings of the National Academy of Sciences, USA* 79(1982):3047–3051.

Estrogens in prevention and treatment of osteoporosis. R. Lindsay. *The Osteoporotic Syndrome: Detection, Prevention, and Treatment,* ed. Avioli, L. V. Orlando, Florida: Grune and Stratton, Inc., 1987, 91–108.

A comparison of mammographic parenchymal patterns in premenopausal Japanese and British women. Gravelle, I. H., R. D. Bulbrook, D. Y. Wang, et al. *Breast Cancer Research and Treatment* 18, suppl (1991):S93–S95.

Effects of alcohol consumption on plasma and urinary hormone concentrations in premenopausal women. Reichman, M. E., J. T. Judd, C. Longcope, et al. *Journal of the National Cancer Institute* 85(1993):722–727.

Estrogen 2-hydroxylase oxidation and menstrual function among elite oarswomen. Snow, R. C., R. L. Barbieri, and R. E. Frisch. *Journal of Clinical Endocrinology and Metabolism* 69(1989):369–376.

Abdominal obesity and breast cancer risk. Schapira, D. V., N. B. Kumar, and G. H. Lyman. *Annals of Internal Medicine* 112(1990):182–186.

Etiology of human breast cancer: a review. MacMahon, B., P. Cole, and J. Brown. *Journal of the National Cancer Institute* 50(1973):21–42.

Sex hormones in women in rural China and in Britain. Key, T. J. A., J. Chen, D. Y. Wang, et al. *British Journal of Cancer* 62(1990):631–636.

Serum hormone levels in pre-menopausal Chinese women in Shanghai and white women in Los Angeles: results from two breast cancer case-control studies. Bernstein, L., J.-M. Yuan, R. K. Ross, et al. *Cancer Causes and Control* 1(1990):51–58.

Chapter Seven

Potential role of tamoxifen in prevention of breast cancer. Nayfield, S. G., J. E. Karp, L. G. Ford, et al. *Journal of the National Cancer Institute* 83(1991):1450–1459.

Prospects for antiestrogen chemoprevention of breast cancer. Love, R. R. *Journal of the National Cancer Institute* 82(1990):18–21.

Tamoxifen as a potential preventive agent in healthy postmenopausal women. Prentice, R. L. *Journal of the National Cancer Institute* 82(1990):1310–1311.

Tamoxifen quandary: promising cancer drug may hide a troubling side. Raloff, J. *Science News* 141(1992):266–269.

Should healthy women take tamoxifen? Fugh-Berman, A. *New England Journal of Medicine* 327(1992):1596–1597.

Breast cancer prevention: hold the hormones, please. Smigel, K. *Journal of the National Cancer Institute* 83(1991):1211–1213.

Induction of covalent DNA adducts in rodents by tamoxifen. Han, X. and J. G. Liehr. *Cancer Research* 52(1992):1360–1363.

LHRH agonists and the prevention of breast and ovarian cancer. Pike, M. C., R. K. Ross, R. A. Lobo, et al. *Lancet* i(1989):142–148.

Concepts in cancer chemopreventive research. Greenwald, P., D. W. Nixon, W. F. Malone, et al. *Cancer* 65(1990):1483–1490.

Chapter Eight

Inhibition of polycyclic aromatic hydrocarbon-induced neoplasia by naturally occurring indoles. Wattenberg, L. W. and W. D. Loub. *Cancer Research* 38(1978):1410–1413.

Inhibition of chemical carcinogenesis. Wattenberg, L. W. *Journal of the National Cancer Institute* 60(1978):11–18.

Effects of dietary indole-3-carbinol on estradiol metabolism and spontaneous mammary tumors in mice. Bradlow, H. L., J. J. Michnovicz, N. T. Telang, et al. *Carcinogenesis* 12(1991):1571–1574.

Induction of estradiol metabolism by dietary indole-3-carbinol in humans. Michnovicz, J. J. and H. L. Bradlow. *Journal of the National Cancer Institute* 82(1990):947–949.

Altered estrogen metabolism and excretion in humans following consumption of indole-3-carbinol. Michnovicz, J. J. and H. L. Bradlow. *Nutrition and Cancer* 16(1991):59–66.

Chemists learn why vegetables are good for you. Angier, N. *The New York Times*, April 13, 1993, C1.

Glucosinolates and their breakdown products in foods and food plants. Fenwick, G. R., R. K. Heaney, and W. J. Mullin. CRC *Critical Reviews of Food Science and Nutrition* 18(1983):123–201.

The role of soy products in reducing risk of cancer. Messina, M. and S. Barnes. *Journal of the National Cancer Institute* 83(1991):541–546.

Nonsteroidal estrogens of dietary origin: possible roles in hormone-dependent disease. Setchell, K. D. R., S. P. Borriello, P. Hulme, et al. *American Journal of Clinical Nutrition* 40(1984):569–578.

Soybeans inhibit mammary tumors in models of breast cancer. Barnes, S., C. Grubbs, and K. D. R. Setchell. *Mutagens and Carcinogens in the Diet*, ed. Pariza, M. New York: Wiley-Liss, Inc., 1990, 239–253.

The Tofu Book. Paino, J. and L. Messinger. Garden City, New York: Avery Publishing Group, 1991.

A prospective study of the intake of vitamins C, E, and A and the risk of breast cancer. Hunter, D. J., J. E. Manson, G. A. Colditz, et al. *New England Journal of Medicine* 329(1993):234–240.

Beyond dietary fiber. Spiller, G. A. *American Journal of Clinical Nutrition* 54(1991):615–617.

Binding of steroid hormones in vitro by water-insoluble dietary fiber. Whitten, C. G. and T. D. Shultz. *Nutrition Research* 8(1988):1223–1235.

High-fiber diet reduces serum estrogen concentrations in premenopausal women. Rose, D. P., M. Goldman, J. M. Connolly, et al. *American Journal of Clinical Nutrition* 54(1991):520–525.

The nutritional incidence of flavonoids: some physiological and metabolic considerations. Roger, C. R., *Experientia* 44(1988):725–804.

Western diet and western diseases: some hormonal and biochemical mechanisms and associations. Adlercreutz, H. *Scandinavian Journal of Clinical and Laboratory Investigation* 50, suppl. 201(1990):3–23.

Does fiber-rich food containing animal lignan precursors protect against both colon and breast cancer? An extension of the "fiber hypothesis." Adlercreutz, H. *Gastroenterology* 86(1984):761–764.

Chapter Nine

NCI dietary guidelines: rationale. Butrum, R. R., C. K. Clifford, and E. Lanza. *American Journal of Clinical Nutrition* 48(1988):888–895.

Junk Food, Fast Food, Health Food—What America Eats and Why. Perl, L. New York: Houghton Mifflin/Clarion Books, 1980.

Chapter Ten

U.S., ending dispute, decides what food labels must tell. Burros, M. *The New York Times*, December 3, 1992, A1.

Fighting fat without being a slave to a diet. Brody, J. E. *The New York Times*, November 25, 1992, C8.

Fast food chains move toward healthier choices. Burklow, J. and A. Aubertin. *Journal of the National Cancer Institute* 83(1991):325–326.

Chapter Eleven

Why do so many women have breasts removed needlessly? Kolata, G. *The New York Times*, May 5, 1993, C13.

American Cancer Society guidelines on screening for breast cancer. Dodd, G. D. *Cancer* 69, suppl (1992):1885–1887.

New data revive the debate over mammography before 50. Kolata, G. *The New York Times*, December 16, 1992, C16.

Mammographic screening in asymptomatic women aged 40 years and older. Council on Scientific Affairs. *Journal of the American Medical Association* 261(1989):2535–2542.

INDEX

231